Ion Channels as Marine Drug Ta

Ion Channels as Marine Drug Targets

Editor

Jean-Marc Sabatier

MDPI • Basel • Beijing • Wuhan • Barcelona • Belgrade • Manchester • Tokyo • Cluj • Tianjin

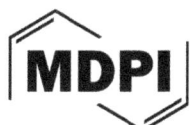

Editor
Jean-Marc Sabatier
Institute of NeuroPhysiopathology
France

Editorial Office
MDPI
St. Alban-Anlage 66
4052 Basel, Switzerland

This is a reprint of articles from the Special Issue published online in the open access journal *Marine Drugs* (ISSN 1660-3397) (available at: https://www.mdpi.com/journal/marinedrugs/special_issues/ion_channels_targets).

For citation purposes, cite each article independently as indicated on the article page online and as indicated below:

LastName, A.A.; LastName, B.B.; LastName, C.C. Article Title. *Journal Name* **Year**, *Volume Number*, Page Range.

ISBN 978-3-03943-797-9 (Hbk)
ISBN 978-3-03943-798-6 (PDF)

Contents

About the Editor

Jean-Marc Sabatier (PhD and HDR) Jean-Marc SABATIER is a Director of research at the French CNRS, with PhD and HDR degrees in Biochemistry and Microbiology. He has led several academic research teams (CNRS, INSERM, and University), as well as a combined academic-industry research laboratory devoted to the engineering of therapeutic peptides (ERT62, Marseilles, France). He was also a Director of Research for several French private companies as well as a Canadian public company. He acts as a Consultant for top pharmaceutical and cosmetic companies. Dr. Sabatier works in the field of animal toxins and microbes. He is the Editor-in-Chief of *Venoms and Toxins*, *Coronaviruses*, and *Infectious Disorders—Drug Targets*. He is also a Topic Editor-in-Chief for *Antibiotics*. He has contributed to several books on toxinology and virology, and more than 160 scientific articles, 180 communications, and 55 patents in both biology and chemistry. He is a member of 60 Editorial Boards of scientific journals, such as *Peptides, Molecules, Antibiotics*, and the *Journal of Biological Chemistry*. He also reviewed articles submitted for publication in 96 international journals and acts as an expert for numerous institutions (ANR, CEA, CNRS, MRC, ISF, BARD, AIRD, IPT, Pasteur Institutes, Ville de Paris, Region Languedoc-Roussillon, Fondation Arthritis, etc.). He won the 'Citizen of the Year Award' from the Nouvel Economiste (1994) for his work on antivirals. He is a member of a dozen scientific societies, such as the 'American Peptide Society' (charter member), 'European Peptide Society', 'American Society for Microbiology', 'Biochemical Society', and 'New-York Academy of Sciences'.

Preface to "Ion Channels as Marine Drug Targets"

Animal venoms, especially of marine origin, are rich natural sources of bioactive compounds. The molecular targets of the latter are mainly ion (i.e., sodium, potassium, calcium, and chloride) channels with their numerous variants/subtypes. These venom molecules are exhibiting diverse potencies and selectivities and may have some therapeutic potential based on their cellular targets. Over the past decade, marine molecules have been widely studied, as they represent potential drugs to treat a variety of (human) pathologies, from pain to autoimmune and neurological diseases. This Special Issue of *Marine Drugs* is devoted to the different aspects of marine (or marine-derived) molecules, from the discovery and structural characterization to the pharmacology and molecular engineering to finally develop some "novel" candidate chemotherapeutic drugs targeting the ion channel(s).

Jean-Marc Sabatier
Editor

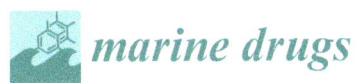

Article

Botulinum Toxin-Chitosan Nanoparticles Prevent Arrhythmia in Experimental Rat Models

David Sergeevichev *, Vladislav Fomenko, Artem Strelnikov, Anna Dokuchaeva, Maria Vasilieva, Elena Chepeleva, Yanina Rusakova, Sergey Artemenko, Alexander Romanov, Nariman Salakhutdinov and Alexander Chernyavskiy

E. Meshalkin National Medical Research Center of the Ministry of Health of the Russian Federation, 15 Rechkunovskaya Str., 630055 Novosibirsk, Russia; vladislav@ngs.ru (V.F.); agstrelnikov@gmail.com (A.S.); a_dokuchaeva@meshalkin.ru (A.D.); vasilievam@yandex.ru (M.V.); e_chepeleva@meshalkin.ru (E.C.); yarojana@mail.ru (Y.R.); s_artemenko@meshalkin.ru (S.A.); abromanov@mail.ru (A.R.); anvar@nioch.nsc.ru (N.S.); amchern@mail.ru (A.C.)
* Correspondence: d_sergeevichev@meshalkin.ru

Received: 2 June 2020; Accepted: 27 July 2020; Published: 2 August 2020

Abstract: Several experimental studies have recently demonstrated that temporary autonomic block using botulinum toxin (BoNT/A1) might be a novel option for the treatment of atrial fibrillation. However, the assessment of antiarrhythmic properties of BoNT has so far been limited, relying exclusively on vagal stimulation and rapid atrial pacing models. The present study examined the antiarrhythmic effect of specially formulated BoNT/A1-chitosan nanoparticles (BTN) in calcium chloride-, barium chloride- and electrically induced arrhythmia rat models. BTN enhanced the effect of BoNT/A1. Subepicardial injection of BTN resulted in a significant antiarrhythmic effect in investigated rat models. BTN formulation antagonizes arrhythmia induced by the activation of Ca, K and Na channels.

Keywords: botulinum toxin A1; chitosan nanoparticles; antiarrhythmics; pharmacological models of arrhythmia; electrically induced arrhythmia

1. Introduction

Botulinum toxin (BoNT) is a safe and efficient therapeutic means to treat a variety of conditions characterized by the hyperfunction of nerve terminals [1,2]. Recently, there has been a growing interest in BoNT for the treatment of atrial fibrillation (AF). Initially, Tsuboi et al. [3] demonstrated that BoNT injected into the sinoatrial fat pad inhibited a decrease in sinus rate in response to vagus nerve stimulation and suggested that BoNT can inhibit ganglionic neurotransmission in the dog heart in situ. Later, Oh et al. [4] demonstrated that direct injection of BoNT in epicardial fat pads temporally suppressed AF inducibility in dogs. In the first clinical study of BoNT effects on patients undergoing coronary artery bypass surgery, Pokushalov et al. [5] demonstrated that BoNT injection suppresses postoperative atrial fibrillation. Recently, Lo et al. [6] demonstrated that suppression of the four major atrial ganglionated plexi by BoNT may break the vicious cycle of "AF begets AF" by inhibiting autonomic remodeling, and possibly preventing subsequent progression of AF to more persistent forms. In addition, Nazeri et al. [7] found that after one week following injection of BoNT into the atrial fat pads of sheep, the vulnerability of atrial tissue to AF induction and the vagal influence on the atrial effective refractory period were reduced compared to baseline levels.

However, the assessment of antiarrhythmic properties of BoNT has only been studied using experimental models of vagal stimulation [3,4,7] and rapid atrial pacing [6]. Indeed, although the effect of BoNT on atrial arrhythmias has attracted much attention, the effects of BoNT on ventricular arrhythmias remain unknown.

Therapeutic doses of botulinum neurotoxin drugs are safe, and side effects are relatively rare. Adverse effects often depend on the injection site: there are skin rash, muscle weakness, fatigue, flu-like symptoms, a dry mouth and dizziness [8]. However, in the "first-in-human" study of the epicardial fat pad botulinum toxin injection for atrial fibrillation prevention, there was no serious adverse effect during the one-year and three-year follow-up period [5,9].

The BoNT block of neuromuscular transmission occurs after a lapse of time [7,10,11] and the blocking effect is temporary, with recovery of neuromuscular transmission within one to six months in skeletal muscles [12] and within three weeks in the heart [4]. Therefore, new formulations that may accelerate the effect of BoNT and increase its duration time are highly desirable. Recently, we have demonstrated that globular chitosan prolongs the block of neuromuscular transmission after the BoNT intramuscular injection in rats [13]. Chitosan is a linear polymer derived from chitin, the second most abundant aminopolysaccharide after cellulose. It is fully biocompatible, studied in numerous pharmaceutical and medical applications, demonstrating the highest possible safety profile [14]. To overcome the poor solubility of linear chitosan in water, we used an improved globular chitosan, Novochizol. Novochizol synthesis comprises a two-step activation of linear chitosan, an intramolecular reaction that cross-links linear chitosan molecules. After the cross-linking procedure, Novochizol can be impregnated with active pharmaceutical ingredients [15].

Therefore, in the present study, we examined the antiarrhythmic effect of BoNT and its formulation with an enhanced globular chitosan (Botulinum_Novochizol, BTN) using calcium chloride-, barium chloride- and electrically induced arrhythmia rat models.

2. Results

Normal ECG waves with a sinus rhythm were observed in all investigated models before intravenous or subepicardial injection of test substances and before injection of arrhythmogens.

2.1. Calcium Chloride-Induced Arrhythmia

Intravenous injection of calcium chloride (150 mg/kg) caused severe lethal ventricular fibrillation (VF) after a few seconds p.i (Table 1, Figure 1). Neither BoNT/A1 intravenous or subepicardial injection nor subepicardial injection of chitosan nanoparticles prevented lethal VF. Subepicardial injection of BoNT/A1 lead to a slight, statistically insignificant increase in the onset time of VF (24.4 ± 2.1 s in the BoNT/A1 group vs. 8.2 ± 1.7 s in the control group, $p = 0.288$). Subepicardial BTN injection prevented lethal VF in five rats and led to a significant increase in the onset time of VF (208.6 ± 46.6 s in the BTN group vs. 8.2 ± 1.7 s in the control group, $p < 0.001$). However, verapamil was more effective than BTN and prevented lethal VF in eight animals, with an initial onset time of VF of 300.0 ± 30.0 s ($p = 0.0000$ vs. control, $p = 0.002$ vs. BTC group). Only rats demonstrating VF were included in the statistical analysis of the initial onset time of VF: there were 10 animals in the control, BoNT/A1 (i.v. and subepicardial) and chitosan nanoparticles groups, two animals in the verapamil group and five animals in the BTN group (Figure 1).

Table 1. The effects of test substances on $CaCl_2$-induced arrhythmia incidence in anesthetized rats.

Test Substances	Sinus Rhythm	Lethal VF	PVC *, Bigeminy, Not VF	The Incidence of VF, *p* (vs. Saline Control, Fisher's Exact Test)
Saline control	0	10	0	
Verapamil	8	2	0	<0.001
BoNT/A1, i.v.	0	10	0	
BoNT/A1, subepicardially	0	10	0	
globular chitosan, subepicardially	0	10	0	
BTN, subepicardially	3	5	2	<0.05

* PVC—premature ventricular contractions.

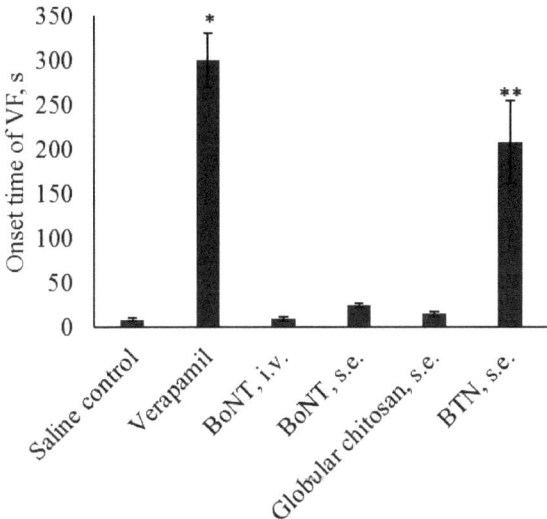

Figure 1. The initial onset time of ventricular fibrillation (VF) after injection of the different tested substances, in the calcium chloride model of arrhythmia. N = 10 for saline, BoNT (intravenously and subepicardially) and chitosan nanoparticle groups, n = 2 for Verapamil group and n = 5 for BTN group (see Table 1). * p < 0.01 vs. control, ** p < 0.01 vs. Verapamil, ANOVA with LSD post hoc test.

Due to all the tested substances, only BTN displayed a significant antiarrhythmic effect 15 min after subepicardial injection, and only this formulation was chosen for further study.

2.2. Barium Chloride-Induced Arrhythmia

Intravenous injection of barium chloride (7.5 mg/kg) caused premature ventricular contractions (PVC), followed by bigeminy 1–5 min after injection, followed by restoration of sinus rhythm. None of the animals perished.

In comparison with the **saline** control, subepicardial BTN injection significantly reduced the incidence of ventricular arrhythmias at doses between 0.5 and 5 U(BoNT/A1)/kg (Table 2). Unexpectedly, a 0.5 U(BoNT/A1)/kg dose proved more effective than 1 and 2 U/kg doses; however, these differences were not significant (p = 0.63 and 0.35, respectively).

Table 2. The effects of test substances on arrhythmia incidence in anesthetized rats, BaCl2-induced arrhythmia.

Test Substances	Sinus Rhythm	Arrhythmia (PVC, Bigeminy)	p (vs. Saline Control, Fisher's Exact Test, Two-Tailed)
Saline control	0	10	
amiodarone	10	0	<0.001
BTN, subepicardially			
0.5 U(BoNT/A1)/kg	8	2	<0.001
1 U(BoNT/A1)/kg	4	6	<0.05
2 U(BoNT/A1)/kg	5	5	<0.05
4 U(BoNT/A1)/kg	8	2	<0.001
5 U(BoNT/A1)/kg	8	2	<0.001

2.3. Electrical Stimulation

There were no statistically significant differences between the values of VFT_0 (threshold of ventricular fibrillation before BTN or lidocaine injection) in different groups. Subepicardial BTN injection increased VFT_1 (threshold of ventricular fibrillation after BTN or lidocaine injection) in a dose-dependent manner (Figure 2). VFT (ventricular fibrillation threshold) was increased by 12% and 10% upon administration of 1 and 2 U(BoNT/A1)/kg, respectively. These differences were not statistically significant. In contrast, VFT was significantly increased by 18% and 20%, upon administration of 4 and 5 U(BoNT/A1)/kg, respectively ($p = 0.0136$ and 0.0177, respectively). The reference antiarrhythmic lidocaine increased the VFT by 13% ($p = 0.0344$).

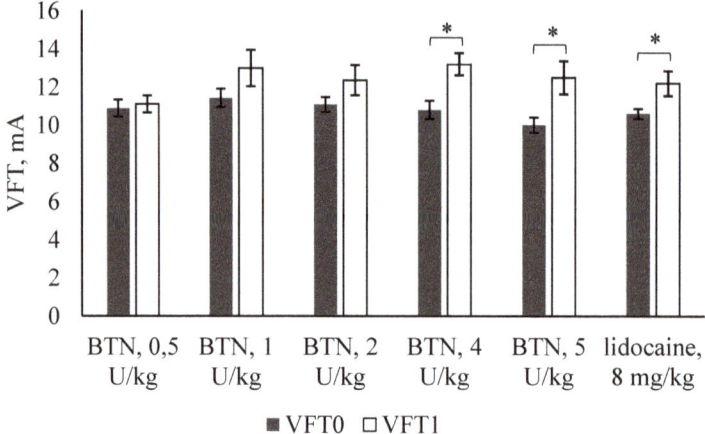

Figure 2. The effect of BTN (subepicardial injection) or lidocaine (i.v.) on VFT in anesthetized rats. VFT_0—minimum electrical intensity that generated VF before injection of BTN or lidocaine; VFT_1—minimum electrical intensity that produced VF after injection of BTN or lidocaine; mean ± SEM (* $p < 0.05$ VFT_1 vs. VFT_0; ANOVA with LSD post hoc test).

3. Discussion

Several studies have shown that temporary autonomic block using BoNT might be a novel therapeutic option for the treatment of postoperative AF [4–6,16]. It is well known that BoNT acts on neuromuscular junctions and blocks the exocytotic release of acetylcholine (ACh) stored in synaptic vesicles [17]. ACh is the main neurotransmitter of the parasympathetic nervous system and an internal transmitter of the sympathetic nervous system [18]. The role of the sympathetic and parasympathetic nervous system in the pathophysiology of cardiac arrhythmias is complex [19]. Selective ablation or stimulation of the different components of the autonomic nervous system, such as ganglionic plexi or the vagal nerve, can modulate the activity of this system and treat arrhythmias [20,21]. By blocking ACh release from the autonomic nerve terminals, BoNT can affect the parasympathetic control of the sinoatrial and atrioventricular node of the heart through the vagal nerve [3,4,22,23].

The antiarrhythmic effects of BoNT injection into ganglionated plexi have been shown to persist for at least one year after cardiac surgery [5,16]. However, it is important to find a way to enhance and further prolong this therapeutic effect. Indeed, patients developing new-onset postoperative atrial fibrillation have a high risk of recurrent atrial fibrillation for as long as two years after surgery [24,25]. Recently, we have demonstrated through intramuscular injection in rats [13] that globular chitosan prolongs the effect of BoNT/A1 and decreases its subsequent toxicity. The persistence of this effect on BoNT/A1 will be investigated in a future study. Here, we assessed the influence of globular (nanoprticle) chitosan on the antiarrhythmic properties of BoNT/A1.

Chitosan is a natural polymer known for its lack of toxicity and immunogenicity, its biodegradability and antimicrobial properties. As such, it is an excellent candidate for a variety of medical and pharmaceutical applications [26,27]. Thanks to their globular form and a high degree of diacylation and in contrast to linear chitosan, globular chitosan used previously [28] and the improved chitosan nanoparticles used in the present study (Novochizol) yield aqueous suspensions equivalent to bona fide solutions. This characteristic is essential for subepicardial or intravenous injection as a clinical application of this compound. As demonstrated in the chloride calcium-induced model of arrhythmia, chitosan nanoparticles alone did not display any antiarrhythmic or arrhythmogenic properties. Thus, the antiarrhythmic effect of BTN is due to the action of BoNT. Accordingly, the dose of BTN was measured as U(BoNT)/kg.

No good model of arrhythmia exists that brings together all the essential anatomopathological, electrophysiological, biochemical and molecular factors present in clinical practice [29]. In addition, the assessment of antiarrhythmic properties of BoNT has relied exclusively on experimental models of vagal stimulation [3,4,7] and rapid atrial pacing [6]. In the present work, we used calcium chloride, barium chloride and left ventricle electrical stimulation to devise three different experimental models of arrhythmia in rats. Intravenous infusion of calcium chloride induces ventricular arrhythmias in animals by increasing intracellular free calcium and opening calcium channels [30]. In contrast, barium chloride decreases outward potassium currents [31]. The influence of the drug on K and Na channels could be assessed in the model of electrical stimulation [32]. Protection against rhythm disturbances caused by these arrhythmogenic factors demonstrates the ability of a compound to act as a potential antiarrhythmic agent.

Intravenous injection is a conventional route of administration for antiarrhythmics used in clinics. Accordingly, we initially administered BoNT/A1 by intravenous injections. However, this mode of administration did not prevent the induced arrhythmias. Instead, antiarrhythmic effects (non-significant for BoNT and statistically significant for BTN) were observed when BoNT/A1 and BTN were injected subepicardially, 15 min before the injection of calcium chloride. One of the limitations in the chosen rat model is the quasi-impossibility to perform an injection in autonomic ganglia or fat pads or even in the wall of the left atrium. Indeed, although the density of small fibers and ganglia is the highest in the posterior part of the left atrium and around the antrum of the pulmonary veins [33,34], the rat's heart is very small and the heart rate is very high. In addition, a dense network of Ach-containing nerves running over the epi- and endocardial surfaces of left and right ventricles and a widespread distribution of muscarinic ACh receptors throughout the ventricle have been demonstrated in different species [35–41]. Therefore, we injected the tested substances subepicardially, in the left ventricles.

Since a time-lapse is required for BoNT to block neuromuscular transmission [7,10,11], we injected BoNT/A1 or BTN 15 min before the injection of arrhythmogens. Our results in the calcium chloride model demonstrated that this delay was not sufficient for BoNT/A1 to show significant antiarrhythmic effects. In contrast, BTN demonstrated clear antiarrhythmic effects despite the short time-lapse between the injection of BTN and the injection of the arrhythmogen. At the same time, chitosan nanoparticles alone did not show antiarrhythmic effect. Therefore, we conclude that chitosan nanoparticles accelerate the effect of BoNT/A1. As the next step, we examined the dose-dependency of BTN effects on the incidence of arrhythmias in either a barium chloride model or after electrical myocardial stimulation of the left ventricle.

There were no significant differences between the antiarrhythmic effect at different doses of BTN (0.5–5 U(BoNT)/kg) in the barium chloride model. Instead, all dosages significantly prevented arrhythmias as compared to the control group. On the other hand, there was a clear dose-dependent antiarrhythmic effect of BTN in the electrically induced model of arrhythmia. In addition, in this model, the effects of the 4 and 5 U(BoNT)/kg doses were comparable to the effects of lidocaine (8 mg/kg).

Our results demonstrate that the chitosan nanoparticle formulation of BoNT/A1 prevents arrhythmia induced by an activation of Ca, K and Na channels. The mechanism of this effect remains unclear. Further study is needed to understand whether BTN acts on ionic channels directly or whether its effect is mediated by the influence on the autonomic nervous system.

In clinical practice, the use of BoNT or BTN for the treatment of postoperative atrial fibrillation may become a promising alternative to the radiofrequency ablation of ganglionated plexi. Ablation techniques cause permanent destruction of anatomic structures of the heart and may become proarrhythmic [42,43]. At the same time, postoperative arrhythmia has been shown to be a transient phenomenon that generally arises in the first week after an operation [44,45]. Accordingly, the temporary nature of the effect of BoNT and subsequent recovery of conduction of the autonomic nervous system constitute an advantage of the investigated technique. Another beneficial finding is that the injection of BoNT into the ganglionated plexi or a subepicardial injection do not cause permanent injury to the autonomic neurons and myocardium.

4. Materials and Methods

4.1. Test Substances

BoNT/A1 (Xeomin) was purchased from Merz Pharmaceutical Gmbh (Frankfurt am Main, Germany); each vial contained 100 U BoNT/A1.

Chitosan nanoparticles (Novochizol) were provided by Bosti Trading (Nicosia, Cyprus). The average molecular weight of the starting chitosan raw material (Chitoclear by Primex, Siglufjörður, Island) was 450–500 kDa, and the degree of deacetylation was at least 90%. While regular, linear chitosan is insoluble at physiological pH, so chitosan nanoparticles may be suspended in aqueous solutions and the resulting suspension may be assimilated to a solution.

BTN was formulated by dissolving the content of one vial (100 U of BoNT/A1) in 1 mL of a 0.25% suspension of chitosan nanoparticles in physiological saline. The formulation was used as early as after 24 h, and up to 10 days after preparation.

4.2. Animals

Male Wistar rats weighing 410 ± 40 g were provided by the vivarium of the Institute of Cytology and Genetics SB RAS (Novosibirsk, Russian Federation). The animals were housed in the vivarium of «E. Meshalkin National medical research center» of the Ministry of Health of the Russian Federation and were allowed free access to water and commercial laboratory complete food. Prior to the experiment, the animals had an acclimatization period of 14 days. A daily physical examination of the animals was performed in accordance with the regulatory requirements. Animals were blindly randomized into groups immediately prior to performing studies.

The use of animals in this study was approved by the Local Ethics Committee of «E. Meshalkin National medical research center» of the Ministry of Health of the Russian Federation. All parts of the protocol were performed in accordance with the recommendations for proper use and care of laboratory animals (European Communities Council Directive 86/609/CEE) and the principles of the Declaration of Helsinki.

4.3. Anesthesia

To induce anesthesia, rats were administered a subcutaneous injection of atropine (0.01 mg/kg) and were subsequently placed in an anesthesia induction chamber with a continuous supply of air containing sevoflurane (3–5%) (Gas Anesthesia System 21100, Ugo Basile, Gemonio, Italy and Small Animal Ventilator 683, Harvard Apparatus, Holliston, MA, USA). Subsequent to anesthesia, each animal was placed on the operating table, and a 24G peripheral intravenous catheter was inserted into the tail vein. Anesthesia was maintained using intravenous (i.v.) administration of 20 mg/kg sodium thiopental solution every 5–10 min. The same catheter was used for intravenous administration of other medications. Mechanical lung ventilation with indoor air was performed using a Rodent Ventilator device (Ugo Basile, Gemonio, Italy) via a tracheostomy tube with a diameter of 3 mm.

4.4. ECG Analysis

Invasive ECG monitoring was performed with peripheral electrode pads. A standard lead II ECG was recorded throughout the experiments using a Schiller AT-6 electrocardiograph (Schiller, Baar, Switzerland). An ECG recording rate of 50 mm/s was used.

The ventricular ectopic activity was assessed according to the diagnostic criteria advocated by Lambeth Conventions (II) [46]. The ECGs were analyzed to determine the onset of episodes of arrhythmias, including premature ventricular contraction (PVC), bigeminy, ventricular tachycardia (VT) and ventricular fibrillation (VF). VT was defined as PVCs lasting ≥4 beats. VF was defined as rapid, irregular QRS complexes.

4.5. Subepicardial Injections

To perform subepicardial injections, the rats were anesthetized as described above, and subsequently intubated and mechanically ventilated. To access the heart, median sternotomy was performed, with subsequent tissue fixation using fixation devices. The left lung was moved aside to expose the left ventricle, and the tested substances were injected subepicardially using an insulin syringe mounted with a 26G needle. ECG was monitored throughout the entire procedure. After 20 min of observation, the rats were euthanized by insufflation of an excessive volume of carbon dioxide for 15 min.

4.6. Assessment of the Antiarrhythmic Effect

The antiarrhythmic effect of the tested substances was assessed in three different models of arrhythmia (induction by calcium chloride, barium chloride or left ventricle electrical stimulation). The arrhythmogenic dose of calcium chloride and barium chloride was determined in a preliminary study as the smallest dose that induced heart rhythm disorders in 100% of the study animals. Clinically approved antiarrhythmics were used as controls for each model of arrhythmia.

4.7. Calcium Chloride-Induced Arrhythmia

Wistar rats were randomly divided into the following groups, comprising 10 animas each:

Group 1. Saline control (physiological saline, 0.9%);
Group 2. Verapamil, intravenously, 2 µg/kg;
Group 3. BoNT/A1, intravenously, 5 U/kg;
Group 4. BoNT/A1, subepicardially, 5 U/kg;
Group 5. Chitosan nanoparticles, subepicardially, 0.014 mg/kg;
Group 6. BTN, subepicardially, 5 U(BoNT/A1)/kg.

Arrhythmia was induced by the intravenous injection of 10% $CaCl_2$ solution (Moschimpharmpreparaty, Moscow, Russian Federation) to reach a final dose of 150 mg/kg. The reference antiarrhythmic verapamil (Ozon, Samara, Russian Federation) was injected intravenously 5 min before the arrhythmogen. Each control rat received 0.1 mL saline 5 min before the injection of the arrhythmogen. Test substances (BoNT/A1, globular chitosan and BTN) were injected intravenously or subepicardially 15 min before the arrhythmogen.

4.8. Barium Chloride-Induced Arrhythmia

The following groups of animals, comprising 10 animas each, were investigated:

Group 1. Saline control (physiological saline, 0.9%);
Group 2. Amiodarone, 5 mg/kg;
Groups 3 to 7. Subepicardial injection of BTN (0.5, 1, 2, 4 and 5 U(BoNT/A1)/kg).

Arrhythmia was induced by an intravenous administration of 2% $BaCl_2$ solution to reach a final dose of 7.5 mg/kg. The $BaCl_2$ stock solution was prepared by dissolving 2 g of $BaCl_2$ (Sigma-Aldrich, St. Louis, MO, USA) in 100 mL of physiological saline under aseptic conditions, and when no particulate matter was visible, the solution was sterilized by passing through a 0.1 μm syringe filter (Millipore, Burlington, MA, USA).

Amiodarone (Sanofi-Aventis, Paris, France) was used as a reference antiarrhythmic and was injected intravenously 5 min before $BaCl_2$. Physiological saline was injected into the control rats 5 min before $BaCl_2$. BTN was injected subepicardially 15 min before $BaCl_2$.

4.9. Electrical Stimulation

Anesthetized rats were subjected to a thoracotomy and left ventricle electrical stimulation using two stainless steel stimulating electrodes. A pacing system analyzer (ERA 300, Biotronik, Lake Oswego, OR, USA) was used to deliver electrical rectangular impulses (pulse-width 5 m, frequency 16.6 Hz). Electrical intensity was initially set at 10 mA and increased in stepwise increments of 1 mA until VF was observed. This minimum electrical intensity that produced VF was set as the threshold current for induction of VF (VF threshold—VFT).

Six groups of animals were investigated, each group comprising 10 animals. VFT_0 was recorded after thoracotomy but before BTN injection. Then, recovery of heart rhythm was observed for 10 min, followed by subepicardial injection of BTN or i.v. injection of lidocaine. VFT_1 was recorded 15 min after injection of BTN (0.5, 1, 2, 4 or 5 U(BoNT/A1)/kg) or lidocaine (8 mg/kg).

4.10. Statistical Analysis

Statistical analyses were carried out using Statistica 13 (TIBCO Software, Palo Alto, CA, USA). Differences were considered significant when $p < 0.05$. The incidences of VF or arrhythmias ($CaCl_2$ or $BaCl_2$ models, respectively) were compared using two-tailed Fisher's exact test.

The onset times of VF (calcium chloride model) and VFT (electrically induced arrhythmia) were expressed as mean ± standard error of the mean (SEM). ANOVA with LSD post hoc test was implemented to identify significant differences between groups.

Author Contributions: Conceptualization, D.S. and A.R.; methodology, D.S., V.F., A.S.; software, M.V.; validation, D.S.; formal analysis, M.V.; investigation, A.D., V.F., E.C., Y.R.; resources, Y.R.; data curation, M.V.; writing—original draft preparation, D.S.; writing—review and editing, N.S., S.A.; visualization, D.S.; project administration, A.C. All authors have read and agreed to the published version of the manuscript.

Funding: This research received no external funding.

Conflicts of Interest: The authors declare no conflict of interest.

References

1. Ramirez-Castaneda, J.; Jankovic, J. Long-term efficacy, safety, and side effect profile of botulinum toxin in dystonia: A 20-year follow-up. *Toxicon* **2014**, *90*, 344–348. [CrossRef]
2. Wheeler, A.; Smith, H.S. Botulinum toxins: Mechanisms of action, antinociception and clinical applications. *Toxicology* **2013**, *306*, 124–146. [CrossRef] [PubMed]
3. Tsuboi, M.; Furukawa, Y.; Kurogouchi, F.; Nakajima, K.; Hirose, M.; Chiba, S. Botulinum neurotoxin A blocks cholinergic ganglionic neurotransmission in the dog heart. *Jpn. J. Pharm.* **2002**, *89*, 249–254. [CrossRef] [PubMed]
4. Oh, S.; Choi, E.K.; Zhang, Y.; Mazgalev, T.N. Botulinum toxin injection in epicardial autonomic ganglia temporarily suppresses vagally mediated atrial fibrillation. *Circ. Arrhythmia Electrophysiol.* **2011**, *4*, 560–565. [CrossRef] [PubMed]

5. Pokushalov, E.; Kozlov, B.; Romanov, A.; Strelnikov, A.; Bayramova, S.; Sergeevichev, D.; Bogachev-Prokophiev, A.; Zheleznev, S.; Shipulin, V.; Lomivorotov, V.V.; et al. Long-term suppression of atrial fibrillation by botulinum toxin injection into epicardial fat pads in patients undergoing cardiac surgery: One-year follow-up of a randomized pilot study. *Circ. Arrhythmia Electrophysiol.* **2015**, *8*, 1334–1341. [CrossRef] [PubMed]
6. Lo, L.W.; Scherlag, B.J.; Chang, H.Y.; Lin, Y.J.; Chen, S.A.; Po, S.S. Temporary suppression of cardiac ganglionated plexi leads to long-term suppression of atrial fibrillation: Evidence of early autonomic intervention to break the vicious cycle of "AF begets AF". *J. Am. Heart Assoc.* **2016**, *5*, e003309. [CrossRef]
7. Nazeri, A.; Ganapathy, A.V.; Massumi, A.; Massumi, M.; Tuzun, E.; Stainback, R.; Segura, A.M.; Elayda, M.A.; Razavi, M. Effect of botulinum toxin on inducibility and maintenance of atrial fibrillation in ovine myocardial tissue. *Pacing Clin. Electrophysiol.* **2017**, *40*, 693–702. [CrossRef]
8. Bakheit, A.M. The possible adverse effects of intramuscular botulinum toxin injections and their management. *Curr. Drug Saf.* **2006**, *1*, 271–279. [CrossRef]
9. Romanov, A.; Pokushalov, E.; Ponomarev, D.; Bayramova, S.; Shabanov, V.; Losik, D.; Stenin, I.; Elesin, D.; Mikheenko, I.; Strelnikov, A.; et al. Long-term suppression of atrial fibrillation by botulinum toxin injection into epicardial fat pads in patients undergoing cardiac surgery: Three-year follow-up of a randomized study. *Heart Rhythm* **2019**, *16*, 172–177. [CrossRef]
10. Kumar, R.; Kukreja, R.V. The Botulinum Toxin as a Therapeutic Agent: Molecular Structure and Mechanism of Action in Motor and Sensory Systems. *Semin. Neurol.* **2016**, *36*, 10–19. [CrossRef]
11. Lebeda, F.J.; Cer, R.Z.; Stephens, R.M.; Mudunuri, U. Temporal characteristics of botulinum neurotoxin therapy. *Expert Rev. Neurother.* **2010**, *10*, 93–103. [CrossRef] [PubMed]
12. Rossetto, O.; Seveso, M.; Caccin, P.; Schiavo, G.; Montecucco, C. Tetanus and botulinum neurotoxins: Turning bad guys into good by research. *Toxicon* **2001**, *39*, 27–41. [CrossRef]
13. Sergeevichev, D.S.; Krasilnikova, A.A.; Strelnikov, A.G.; Fomenko, V.V.; Salakhutdinov, N.F.; Romanov, A.B.; Karaskov, A.M.; Pokushalov, E.A.; Steinberg, J.S. Globular chitosan prolongs the effective duration time and decreases the acute toxicity of botulinum neurotoxin after intramuscular injection in rats. *Toxicon* **2018**, *143*, 90–95. [CrossRef] [PubMed]
14. Khan, M.I.H.; An, X.; Dai, L.; Li, H.; Khan, A.; Ni, Y. Chitosan-based Polymer Matrix for Pharmaceutical Excipients and Drug Delivery. *Curr. Med. Chem.* **2019**, *26*, 2502–2513. [CrossRef]
15. Novochizol First-In-Class Polysaccharide Nanotechnology Home Page. Available online: https://www.novochizol.ch/what/ (accessed on 21 July 2020).
16. Pokushalov, E.; Kozlov, B.; Romanov, A.; Strelnikov, A.; Bayramova, S.; Sergeevichev, D.; Bogachev-Prokophiev, A.; Zheleznev, S.; Shipulin, V.; Lomivorotov, V.V.; et al. Botulinum toxin injection in epicardial fat pads can prevent recurrences of atrial fibrillation after cardiac surgery: Results of a randomized pilot study. *J. Am. Coll. Cardiol.* **2014**, *64*, 628–629. [CrossRef]
17. Schiavo, G.; Montecucco, C. Clostridial Neurotoxins. In *Bacterial Toxins: Tools in Cell Biology and Pharmacology*; Aktories, K., Ed.; John Wiley & Sons: Hoboken, NJ, USA, 2008; pp. 169–192.
18. Roy, A.; Guatimosim, S.; Prado, V.F.; Gros, R.; Prado, M.A.M. Cholinergic activity as a new target in diseases of the heart. *Mol. Med.* **2015**, *20*, 527–537. [CrossRef]
19. Krul, S.P.J.; Berger, W.R.; Veldkamp, M.W.; Driessen, A.H.G.; Wilde, A.A.M.; Deneke, T.; de Bakker, J.M.T.; Coronel, R.; de Groot, J.R. Treatment of Atrial and Ventricular Arrhythmias through Autonomic Modulation. *JACC Clin. Electrophysiol.* **2015**, *1*, 496–508. [CrossRef]
20. Katritsis, D.G.; Pokushalov, E.; Romanov, A.; Giazitzoglou, E.; Siontis, G.C.M.; Po, S.S.; Camm, A.J.; Ioannidis, J.P.A. Autonomic denervation added to pulmonary vein isolation for paroxysmal atrial fibrillation: A randomized clinical trial. *J. Am. Coll. Cardiol.* **2013**, *62*, 2318–2325. [CrossRef]
21. Parwani, P.; Abbas, M.; Filiberti, A.; Fleming, C.; Hu, Y.; Garabelli, P.; Mcunu, A.; Peyton, M.; Po, S.S. Low-level vagus nerve stimulation suppresses post-operative atrial fibrillation and inflammation: A randomized study. *JACC Clin. Electrophysiol.* **2017**, *3*, 929–938. [CrossRef]
22. Dickson, E.C.; Shevky, R. Botulism. Studies on the manner in which the toxin of clostridium botulinum acts upon the body: The effect upon the autonomic nervous system. *J. Exp. Med.* **1923**, *37*, 711–731. [CrossRef]
23. Mehnert, U.; de Kort, L.M.; Wöllner, J.; Kozomara, M.; van Koeveringe, G.A.; Kessler, T.M. Effects of onabotulinumtoxinA on cardiac function following intradetrusor injections. *Exp. Neurol.* **2016**, *285*, 167–172. [CrossRef] [PubMed]

24. Lomivorotov, V.V.; Efremov, S.M.; Pokushalov, E.A.; Karaskov, A.M. New-onset atrial fibrillation after cardiac surgery: Pathophysiology, prophylaxis, and treatment. *J. Cardiothorac. Vasc. Anesth.* **2016**, *30*, 200–216. [CrossRef] [PubMed]

25. Lomivorotov, V.V.; Efremov, S.M.; Pokushalov, E.A.; Romanov, A.B.; Ponomarev, D.N.; Cherniavsky, A.M.; Shilova, A.N.; Karaskov, A.M.; Lomivorotov, V.N. Randomized trial of fish oil infusion to prevent atrial fibrillation after cardiac surgery: Data from an implantable continuous cardiac monitor. *J. Cardiothorac. Vasc. Anesth.* **2014**, *28*, 1278–1284. [CrossRef] [PubMed]

26. Cheung, R.C.F.; Ng, T.B.; Wong, J.H.; Chan, W.Y. Chitosan: An update on potential biomedical and pharmaceutical applications. *Mar. Drugs* **2015**, *13*, 5156–5186. [CrossRef]

27. Kato, Y.; Onishi, H.; Machida, Y. Application of chitin and chitosan derivatives in the pharmaceutical field. *Curr. Pharm. Biotechnol.* **2003**, *4*, 303–309. [CrossRef]

28. Krasilnikova, A.A.; Sergeevichev, D.S.; Fomenko, V.V.; Korobeynikov, A.A.; Vasilyeva, M.B.; Yunoshev, A.S.; Karaskov, A.M.; Pokushalov, E.A. Globular chitosan treatment of bovine jugular veins: Evidence of anticalcification efficacy in the subcutaneous rat model. *Cardiovasc. Pathol.* **2018**, *32*, 1–7. [CrossRef]

29. Chorro, F.J.; Such-Belenguer, L.; López-Merino, V. Animal models of cardiovascular disease. *Rev. Esp. Cardiol.* **2009**, *62*, 69–84. [CrossRef]

30. Barzu, T.; Dam, D.T.; Cuparencu, B.; Komendat, M.; Szasz, E. An analysis of calcium chloride-induced arrhythmias in rats. *Agressologie* **1978**, *19*, 293–298.

31. Czopek, A.; Byrtus, H.; Zagorska, A.; Siwek, A.; Kazek, G.; Dudnarski, M.; Sapa, J.; Pawlowski, M. Design, synthesis, anticonvulsant, and antiarrhythmic properties of novel N-Mannich base and amide derivatives of b-tetralinohydantoin. *Pharm. Rep.* **2016**, *68*, 886–893. [CrossRef]

32. Pugsley, M.K.; Hayes, E.S.; Wang, W.Q.; Walker, M.J.A. Ventricular arrhythmia incidence in the rat is reduced by naloxone. *Pharm. Res.* **2015**, *97*, 64–69. [CrossRef]

33. Chevalier, P.; Tabib, A.; Meyronnet, D.; Chalabreysse, L.; Restier, L.; Ludman, V.; Alies, A.; Adeleine, P.; Thivolet, F.; Burri, H.; et al. Quantitative study of nerves of the human left atrium. *Heart Rhythm* **2005**, *2*, 518–522. [CrossRef] [PubMed]

34. Tan, A.Y.; Li, H.; Wachsmann-Hogiu, S.; Chen, L.S.; Chen, P.S.; Fishbein, M.C. Autonomic innervation and segmental muscular disconnections at the human pulmonary vein-atrial junction. Implications for catheter ablation of atrial-pulmonary vein junction. *J. Am. Coll. Cardiol.* **2006**, *48*, 132–143. [CrossRef] [PubMed]

35. Batulevicius, D.; Pauziene, N.; Pauza, D.H. Architecture and age-related analysis of the neuronal number of the guinea pig intrinsic cardiac nerve plexus. *Ann. Anat. Anat. Anz.* **2005**, *187*, 225–243. [CrossRef] [PubMed]

36. Kawano, H.; Okada, R.; Yano, K. Histological study on the distribution of autonomic nerves in the human heart. *Heart Vessel.* **2003**, *18*, 32–39. [CrossRef] [PubMed]

37. Pauza, D.H.; Skripka, V.; Pauziene, N.; Stropus, R. Morphology, distribution, and variability of the epicardiac neural ganglionated subplexuses in the human heart. *Anat. Rec.* **2000**, *259*, 353–382. [CrossRef]

38. Rysevaite, K.; Saburkina, I.; Pauziene, N.; Noujaim, S.F.; Jalife, J.; Pauza, D.H. Morphologic pattern of the intrinsic ganglionated nerve plexus in mouse heart. *Heart Rhythm* **2011**, *8*, 448–454. [CrossRef]

39. Rysevaite, K.; Saburkina, I.; Pauziene, N.; Vaitkevicius, R.; Noujaim, S.F.; Jalife, J.; Pauza, D.H. Immunohistochemical characterization of the intrinsic cardiac neural plexus in whole-mount mouse heart preparations. *Heart Rhythm* **2011**, *8*, 731–738. [CrossRef]

40. Saburkina, I.; Rysevaite, K.; Pauziene, N.; Mischke, K.; Schauerte, P.; Jalife, J.; Pauza, D.H. Epicardial neural ganglionated plexus of ovine heart: Anatomic basis for experimental cardiac electrophysiology and nerve protective cardiac surgery. *Heart Rhythm* **2010**, *7*, 942–950. [CrossRef]

41. Ulphani, J.S.; Cain, J.H.; Inderyas, F.; Gordon, D.; Gikas, P.V.; Shade, G.; Mayor, D.; Arora, R.; Kadish, A.H.; Goldberger, J.J. Quantitative analysis of parasympathetic innervation of the porcine heart. *Heart Rhythm* **2010**, *7*, 1113–1119. [CrossRef]

42. Buckley, U.; Rajendran, P.S.; Shivkumar, K. Ganglionated plexus ablation for atrial fibrillation: Just because we can, does that mean we should? *Heart Rhythm* **2017**, *14*, 133–134. [CrossRef]

43. Lo, L.W.; Scherlag, B.J.; Chang, H.Y.; Lin, Y.J.; Chen, S.A.; Po, S.S. Paradoxical long-term proarrhythmic effects after ablating the head station ganglionated plexi of the vagal innervation to the heart. *Heart Rhythm* **2013**, *10*, 751–757. [CrossRef] [PubMed]

44. Aranki, S.F.; Shaw, D.P.; Adams, D.H.; Rizzo, R.J.; Couper, G.S.; VanderVliet, M.; Collins, J.J.; Cohn, L.H.; Burstin, H.R. Predictors of atrial fibrillation after coronary artery surgery: Current trends and impact on hospital resources. *Circulation* **1996**, *94*, 390–397. [CrossRef] [PubMed]
45. Rostagno, C.; Blanzola, C.; Pinelli, F.; Rossi, A.; Carone, E.; Stefano, P.L. Atrial fibrillation after isolated coronary surgery. Incidence, long term effects and relation with operative technique. *Heart Lung Vessel.* **2014**, *6*, 171–179. [PubMed]
46. Curtis, M.J.; Hancox, J.C.; Farkas, A.; Wainwright, C.L.; Stables, C.L.; Saint, D.A.; Clements-Jewery, H.; Lambiase, P.D.; Billman, G.E.; Janse, M.J.; et al. The Lambeth conventions (II): Guidelines for the study of animal and human ventricular and supraventricular arrhythmias. *Pharm. Ther.* **2013**, *139*, 213–248. [CrossRef] [PubMed]

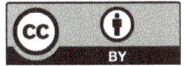

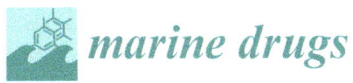 *marine drugs*

Article

Characterisation of δ-Conotoxin TxVIA as a Mammalian T-Type Calcium Channel Modulator

Dan Wang [1], S.W.A. Himaya [1], Jean Giacomotto [2,3], Md. Mahadhi Hasan [1], Fernanda C. Cardoso [1], Lotten Ragnarsson [1] and Richard J. Lewis [1,*]

[1] Institute for Molecular Bioscience, The University of Queensland, Brisbane, QLD 4072, Australia; dan.wang@imb.uq.edu.au (D.W.); h.siddhihalu@imb.uq.edu.au (S.W.A.H.); mahadhi.hasan@imb.uq.edu.au (M.M.H.); f.caldascardoso@imb.uq.edu.au (F.C.C.); l.ragnarsson@imb.uq.edu.au (L.R.)

[2] Queensland Brain Institute, The University of Queensland, Brisbane, QLD 4072, Australia; j.giacomotto@uq.edu.au

[3] Queensland Centre for Mental Health Research, West Moreton Hospital and Health Service and University of Queensland, Brisbane, QLD 4072, Australia

* Correspondence: r.lewis@imb.uq.edu.au; Tel.: +617-3346-2984

Received: 12 May 2020; Accepted: 25 June 2020; Published: 30 June 2020

Abstract: The 27-amino acid (aa)-long δ-conotoxin TxVIA, originally isolated from the mollusc-hunting cone snail *Conus textile*, slows voltage-gated sodium (Na$_V$) channel inactivation in molluscan neurons, but its mammalian ion channel targets remain undetermined. In this study, we confirmed that TxVIA was inactive on mammalian Na$_V$1.2 and Na$_V$1.7 even at high concentrations (10 μM). Given the fact that invertebrate Na$_V$ channel and T-type calcium channels (Ca$_V$3.x) are evolutionarily related, we examined the possibility that TxVIA may act on Ca$_V$3.x. Electrophysiological characterisation of the native TxVIA on Ca$_V$3.1, 3.2 and 3.3 revealed that TxVIA preferentially inhibits Ca$_V$3.2 current (IC$_{50}$ = 0.24 μM) and enhances Ca$_V$3.1 current at higher concentrations. In fish bioassays TxVIA showed little effect on zebrafish behaviours when injected intramuscular at 250 ng/100 mg fish. The binding sites for TxVIA at Na$_V$1.7 and Ca$_V$3.1 revealed that their channel binding sites contained a common epitope.

Keywords: TxVIA; mammalian Na$_V$ channel; selective inhibitor; T-type Ca$_V$3.2

1. Introduction

The δ-conotoxin TxVIA (King Kong peptide), a 27-amino acid (aa)-long peptide with six cysteine residues, was originally isolated from the mollusc-hunting cone snail species *Conus textile* [1]. The unique name of TxVIA, "King Kong peptide", stems from the dominant posture lobsters adopt following injection of the toxin, although it has also been observed to produce convulsive-like activity in snails [1]. TxVIA also produced a paralytic effect in molluscs (*Patella*) but not in fish (*Cambusia*), insects (*Sarcophaga*) or crustaceans (*Porcellio*) [2]. Although no mammalian activity has been reported, TxVIA was shown to potently slow Na$_V$ channel inactivation in molluscs [3]. Previous binding and electrophysiological studies suggest TxVIA binds to both mollusc and rat brain Na$_V$s at sites adjacent to the binding sites of conotoxin CsTx and coral toxin GPT [4–6]. However, TxVIA binding to mammalian Na$_V$ channels is non-functional [4]. The disparate sequence alignment of the *Aplysia* Na$_V$ channel with hNa$_V$1.7 (44% similarity overall, with especially poor overlap across the extracellular regions) supports the distinct modes of action at these distantly related sodium channels.

T-type calcium channels (Ca$_V$3.x) have been identified with two ion-selectivity filters [7], which allow permeability to Na$^+$ ions in the absence of Ca^{2+} ions, with genomic studies on the jellyfish Na$_V$ channel, revealing an ancestral resemblance to Ca$_V$3.x [8]. Ca$_V$3.x provides a privileged gate for calcium influx that initiates many physiological events including secretion, neurotransmission and cell proliferation [9,10], implicating it in many pathophysiological disorders and diseases, including absence epilepsy, Parkinson's disease (PD), hypertension, cardiovascular diseases, cancers and pain [11]. The evolutionary relationship between the invertebrate Na_V channel with $Ca_V3.x$ raised the possibility that TxVIA may modulate $Ca_V3.x$.

In this work, we identified the spatial distribution of TxVIA in the *C. textile* venom duct, isolated and characterised native TxVIA at human $Ca_V3.x$ using Fluorescent Imaging Plate Reader (FLIPR) and electrophysiological (QPatch) assays, confirmed the lack of activity of TxVIA on human Na_V channels endogenously expressed in SH-SY5Y cells [12] and mouse $Na_V1.7$, and used zebrafish [13,14] to analyse behavioural effects using an automated tracking device (i.e. Zebrabox). Finally, we compared the binding sites for TxVIA predicted from molecular docking studies using homology models of $Na_V1.7$ and $Ca_V3.1$.

2. Results

2.1. Distribution, Isolation and Identification of Native TxVIA

C. textile venom ducts of thirteen specimens (TEX-1–13) were dissected into distal (D), distal central (DC), proximal central (PC) and proximal (P) sections, and the extracted venom from each section was analysed by liquid chromatography/mass spectrometry (LC/MS). TxVIA expression across the thirteen specimens (Figure 1a) was localised to the central portions of the *C. textile* venom duct. Guided by TxVIA distribution, the distal central venom of TEX-4 was selected for fractionation (Figure 1b). Native TxVIA was isolated and its amino acid sequence WCKQSGEMCNLLDQNCCDGYCIVLVCT confirmed by tandem mass spectrometry (MS/MS) analysis.

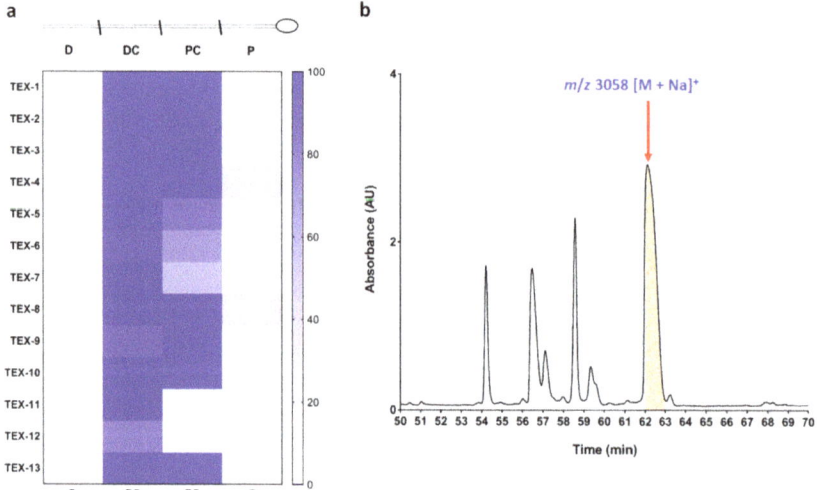

Figure 1. (**a**) TxVIA distribution across the four venom duct sections (distal (D), distal central (DC), proximal central (PC), proximal (P)) of 13 *Conus textile* specimens. (**b**) Partial chromatogram of TEX-4 DC section fractionation. The *x*-axis represents the retention time, the *y*-axis represents UV absorption at 214 nm, and the red arrow indicates TxVIA eluting at 62.5 min (mass data obtained by MALDI-TOF MS).

2.2. Evaluation of Mammalian Na_V Channel Activitiy of TxVIA using FLIPR Cell-Based Assays

TxVIA (5 µM) was tested in SH-SY5Y cells using a FLIPR assay to measure endogenously expressed $Na_V1.2$ and $Na_V1.7$ [12]. Although 0.5 µM TxVIA has previously been shown to slow inactivation of molluscan Na_V current [3], 5 µM TxVIA did not produce any detectable effect on human Na_V responses in SH-SY5Y cells ($n = 3$, $p = 0.37$) (Figure 2a). TxVIA (10 μM) also failed to significantly modify calcium influx in HEK cells transiently expressing mouse $Na_V1.7$ ($n = 2$, $p = 0.29$) (Figure 2b).

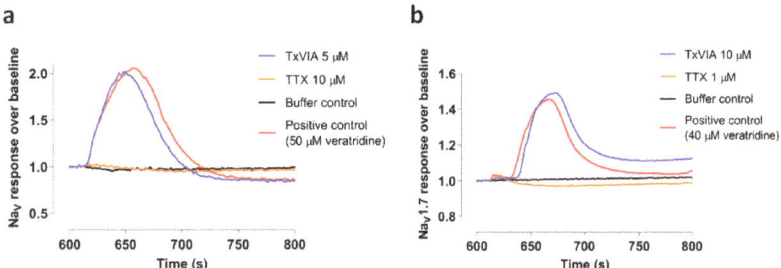

Figure 2. Characterisation of TxVIA in sodium channels. (**a**) Representative fluorescent traces of the hNa_V responses with and without the addition of 5 μM TxVIA. (**b**) Representative fluorescent traces of the mouse $Na_V1.7$ responses with and without the addition of 10 μM TxVIA.

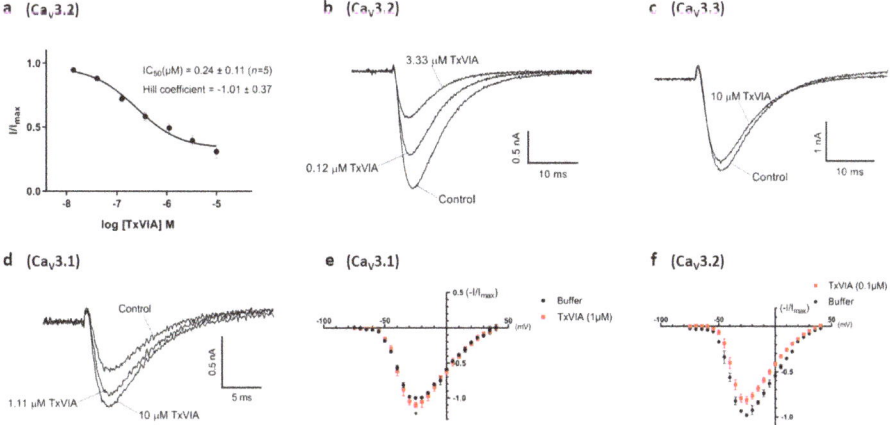

Figure 3. Modulation of $Ca_V3.1$, $Ca_V3.2$ and $Ca_V3.3$ current by TxVIA. (**a**) Concentration response curves of TxVIA on recombinant $hCa_V3.2$ channels ($n = 5$) using the QPatch. Data are means ± SEM. (**b**) Representative $Ca_V3.2$ I_{Ca} during 200 ms depolarisations to V_{max} (−20 mV) from a holding potential of −90 mV before and after perfusions of 0.12 μM and 3.33 μM of TxVIA, as indicated. (**c**) Representative $Ca_V3.3$ I_{Ca} during 200 ms depolarisations to V_{max} (−10 mV) from a holding potential of −90 mV before and after perfusions of 10 μM of TxVIA, as indicated. (**d**) Representative $Ca_V3.1$ I_{Ca} during 200 ms depolarisations to V_{max} (−20 mV) from a holding potential of −90 mV before and after perfusions of 1.11 μM and 10 μM of TxVIA, as indicated. (**e**) Normalised I–V relationships of $Ca_V3.1$ ($n = 5$) plotted from −75 mV to +40 mV before (black) and after (red) the addition of 1 μM of TxVIA, V_{max} at −25 mV (10.0% ± 3.9% current enhancement, $p = 0.04$), I_{max} at 0.12 ± 0.01 nA. Data are means ± SEM. Single-voltage protocol was applied in between to measure the TxVIA effect. (**f**) Normalised I–V relationships of $Ca_V3.2$ ($n = 4$) plotted from −75 mV to +40 mV before (black) and after (red) the addition of 0.1 μM of TxVIA, V_{max} at −25 mV, I_{max} at 0.65 ± 0.04 nA. Data are means ± SEM. Single-voltage protocol was applied in between to measure the TxVIA effect.

2.3. Pharmacological Characterisation of TxVIA in $Ca_V3.x$

We examined the effects of native TxVIA on human $Ca_V3.x$ by whole-cell patch-clamp using the automated electrophysiology platform QPatch 16 X (Figure 3). Whereas TxVIA partially inhibited $Ca_V3.2$ ($n = 5$) (Figure 3a,b) at high nanomolar concentrations, it had little effect on $Ca_V3.3$ ($n = 6$) (Figure 3c) and promoted the opening of $Ca_V3.1$ ($n = 5$) (Figure 3d). Current-voltage (I–V) relationships of Ca$_V$3.1 in the presence of 1 μM TxVIA revealed that the channel modulation was not accompanied by shifts in the *I–V* relationship (*n* = 5, *p* = 0.63) (Figure 3e). Similarly, 0.1 μM TxVIA did not shift the *I–V* relationship of Ca$_V$3.2 (*n* = 4, *p* = 0.21) (Figure 3f). We also tested native TxVIA in the Ca$_V$3.2 FLIPR window current assay [15], where 60 μM TxVIA only showed partial (42%) inhibition (*n* = 3) (data not shown).

2.4. TxVIA Docking in Human Na$_V$1.7 and Ca$_V$3.x

Previous binding and electrophysiological studies have suggested that TxVIA binds to a variety of Na$_V$s despite its lack of functional effects on rat brain Na$_V$s [4], and human Na$_V$1.2 and Na$_V$1.7 responses (present study). The binding site of TxVIA is expected to be extracellular, likely adjacent to but distinct from neurotoxin site 3 [4–6]. Site 3 was initially recognised to be located in the S5-S6 linker of domain I (DI) and IV (DIV) [16], and a later study identified that additional residues in the DIV S3-S4 linker influenced α-scorpion and sea anemone toxin binding [17,18]. Based on this background, we docked TxVIA to the DIV S3-S4 linker of the cryo-electron microscopy (Cryo-EM) structure of human Na$_V$1.7-β1-β2 complex (Protein Data Bank (PDB) code 6J8I) [19]. This docking generated a docking pose where TxVIA fits between the DIV S1-S2 and S3-S4 linkers of Na$_V$1.7 (Figure 4a,b) (Table 1). Importantly, this binding pose identified a strong salt bridge between K3 in TxVIA and E1545 in the DIV S1-S2 linker that is a likely key binding determinant (Figure 4b).

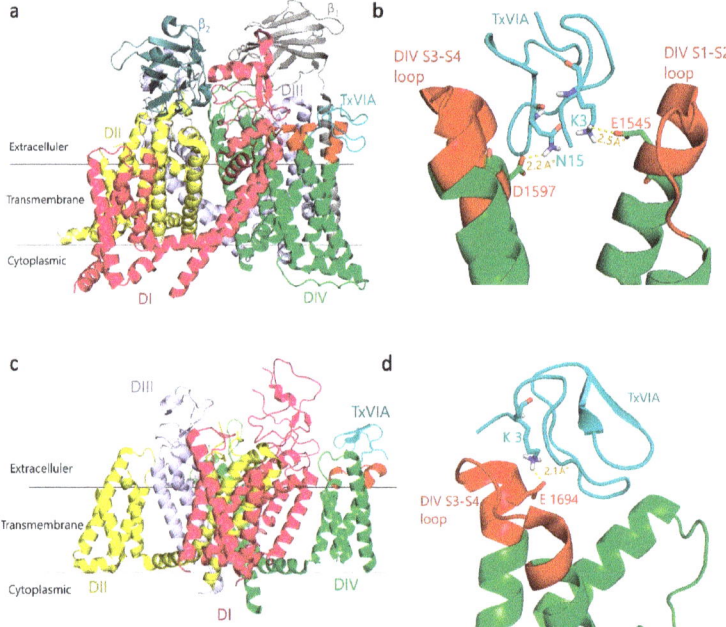

Figure 4. Predicted binding mode of TxVIA (coloured cyan) in human Na$_V$1.7 and Ca$_V$3.1. (**a**) General view of the lowest energy docking pose of TxVIA binding to hNa$_V$1.7 DIV S3-S4 and S1-S2 linkers (extracellular loops, coloured red). (**b**) Local view of TxVIA interactions highlighting that D1597 in hNa$_V$1.7 DIV S3-S4 linker and E1545 in DIV S1-S2 linker make close contact with N15 and K3 of TxVIA, respectively. (**c**) General view of the lowest energy docking pose of TxVIA binding to hCa$_V$3.1 DIV S3-S4 linker (coloured red). (**d**) Local view of the close interaction between K3 in TxVIA and E1694 in the hCa$_V$3.1 DIV S3-S4 linker. Predicted hydrogen bonds are shown as yellow dashed lines, with distances shown in Å.

Table 1. TxVIA binding affinity in human Na$_V$1.7 and Ca$_V$3.x.

Docking Target	Molar Affinity (kcal/mol)
hNa$_V$1.7 DIV S3-S4	−3.2
hNa$_V$1.7 DII S3-S4	7.2
hCa$_V$3.1 DIV S3-S4	−4.0
hCa$_V$3.2 DIV S3-S4	49.1
hCa$_V$3.3 DIV S3-S4	31.8

The 30-aa spider toxin ProTx-II, initially identified as a Na$_V$1.7 selective blocker [20], has also been shown to selectively block the hCa$_V$3.2 current among the three Ca$_V$3.x subtypes [21]. As a well-established site 4 (DII S3-S4 linker) toxin [22], the crystal structure of the ProTx-II-DII hNa$_V$1.7 complex [23] has been generated. It has been suggested that TxVIA binds to a different binding site from ProTx-II [4], which was also supported by our docking results with unfavourable binding affinity (Table 1).

We also explored TxVIA binding in hCa$_V$3.x. The MolProbity score of Ca$_V$3.2 and Ca$_V$3.3 homology models generated from the recently reported hCa$_V$3.1 Cryo-EM structure [24] were 1.97 and 1.98 respectively, indicating the high quality of the modelled structures. An assessment of the Ramachandran plot showed that only 1.85% and 1.34% residues fell in outlier regions for Ca$_V$3.2 and Ca$_V$3.3 models, respectively, with no outliers found for residues in the DIV S3-S4 linker region.

The selective inhibition of ProTx-I [21] for Ca$_V$3.1 current over Ca$_V$3.2 has been identified to be partly attributed to the DIV S3-S4 linker in T-type Ca$_V$s [25]. Interestingly, our docking results also suggest that TxVIA would bind to the DIV S3-S4 linker of Ca$_V$3.1 (Figure 4c,d) with higher affinity than to Ca$_V$3.2 and Ca$_V$3.3 (Table 1). However, the possibility that the DIV S3-S4 linker may contribute to the activation of Ca$_V$3.1 by TxVIA requires further study. Similar to its docking at Na$_V$1.7, the best docking pose for TxVIA binding to Ca$_V$3.1 shows TxVIA interacting between DIV S1-S2 and S3-S4 linkers of Ca$_V$3.1. As shown in Figure 4d, a strong salt bridge was again identified between K3 in TxVIA and E1694 in the Ca$_V$3.1 DIV S3-S4 linker, although no interactions were identified between TxVIA and the S1-S2 in Ca$_V$3.1 DIV.

2.5. Behavioural Analysis on Zebrafish after Intramuscular Injection of TxVIA

Although the TxVIA inhibition of Ca$_V$3.2 indicated possible pain-relieving activity, its activation of Ca$_V$3.1 indicated a possible pain inducing activity, albeit at higher concentrations. We also showed that TxVIA had no effect on the human pain related Na$_V$1.7. Given the potential of TxVIA to play a defensive role, we examined its effect on zebrafish at concentrations up to 250 ng/100 mg fish. However, TxVIA could have different pharmacology on zebrafish and mammalian Ca$_V$s and Na$_V$s that may influence interpretation of responses in zebrafish.

None of the injected fish showed signs indicative of pain-related behaviours or paralysis after the injection ($n = 3$, $p = 0.37$), and no adverse effects were observed in the 24 h post-injection. Fish swimming tracks were also recorded during the first 15 min post-injection (see Figure 5). Zebrafish injected with 250 ng/100 mg fish of TxVIA showed reduced swimming activity compared to control fish in the first 8 min, however this effect did not reach significance and soon reversed to normal edge swimming. Additionally, the absence of swimming bursts or erratic swimming behaviour after TxVIA injection indicates that pain pathways were not activated.

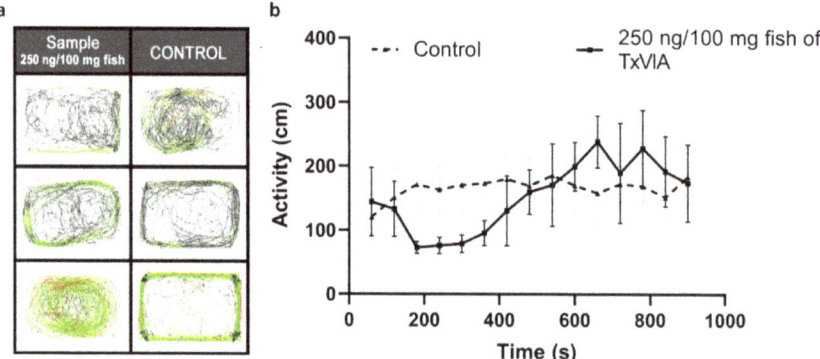

Figure 5. TxVIA-induced behavioural response in adult zebrafish (*n* = 3). (**a**) The six boxes illustrate the 15 min swimming tracks of the control zebrafish (*n* = 3) and the zebrafish injected with 250 ng/100 mg fish of TxVIA (*n* = 3), respectively. The fish generally start with a comparatively slow swimming speed, indicated in black lines, and end with a regular swimming speed, indicated in green lines. Erratic or fast swimming tracks are indicated in red lines. (**b**) The adult zebrafish injected with 250 ng/100 mg fish of TxVIA (continuous line) showed a reduced activity (measured by distance travelled per min) in the first 8 min compared to the activity of the control fish injected with saline sterilised water (dotted line), followed by a small burst of activities for 5 min, and returned to normal gradually. Data are means ± SEM.

3. Discussion

Conotoxins are potent and selective modulators of mammalian ion channels and receptors. The King Kong peptide TxVIA has previously been characterised as a mollusc Na$_V$ channel modulator, producing convulsive-like activity in snails [1] and paralytic effects in the mollusc *Patella* sp. [2]. In this study, we characterised the effects of TxVIA on human Na$_V$s and Ca$_V$3.x, and zebrafish behaviours. These studies revealed for the first time that TxVIA is a nM inhibitor of Ca$_V$3.2 with activating activity on Ca$_V$3.1 at µM concentrations. Interestingly, high concentrations of TxVIA (5 µM) were inactive on endogenously expressed Na$_V$s in SH-SY5Y cells, including Na$_V$1.2 and Na$_V$1.7, or heterologously expressed mouse Na$_V$1.7 (10 µM). In addition, our experiments found that TxVIA does not trigger pain-like behaviours or paralysis in zebrafish at up to 250 ng/100 mg fish, consistent with the lack of an excitatory effect on vertebrate Na$_V$s. Although TxVIA did not target the Ca$_V$3.x window current like Ca$_V$3.x small molecule blockers [26,27], electrophysiological characterisation of TxVIA revealed it to be a nM inhibitor for Ca$_V$3.2 (IC$_{50}$ = 0.24 µM). Ca$_V$3.2 is considered to be a promising novel therapeutic target for pain with Ca$_V$3.2 playing a major pronociceptive role in spinal nociceptive neurons and primary afferents [28–30].

Our LC-MS analysis of dissected *C. textile* venoms revealed that TxVIA was expressed at its highest levels in the central region of the venom duct as the dominant component. Previous studies from our laboratory have revealed that *Conus geographus* and *Conus marmoreus* have evolved to produce defensive and predatory venoms from the proximal and distal regions of the venom duct, respectively, that are deployed in response to the corresponding stimuli [31]. However, the role of central regions of the venom duct in these processes remains unknown. In future studies, we aim to investigate the contribution of TxVIA to the defensive and predatory milked venoms of *C. textile* to unravel its role in defensive and/or predatory behaviour.

To gain insight into TxVIA binding to Na$_V$ and Ca$_V$ channels, we performed molecular docking studies of TxVIA binding to Cryo-EM structures of hNa$_V$1.7 and hCa$_V$3.1. A strong salt bridge was identified in TxVIA binding to the DIV S1-S2 linker of Na$_V$1.7, suggesting that the DIV S1-S2 linker could be a new binding site affecting Na$_V$ channel targeting neurotoxins. Our docking studies of TxVIA in hCa$_V$3.x showed that TxVIA binds to the DIV S3-S4 linker of Ca$_V$3.1 with a strong salt bridge, whereas it failed to dock to the DIV S3-S4 linker of Ca$_V$3.2 and Ca$_V$3.3. These results suggested that the interaction sites between TxVIA and hCa$_V$3.x may differ among the three subtypes, which is supported by our electrophysiological data showing it has differential effects across the three subtypes. We speculate that the DIV S3-S4 linker may contribute to both the selective inhibition [25] and activation of the Ca$_V$3.1 current.

Toxins with the inhibitor cystine knot (ICK) motif have been mostly recognised as modulators of voltage-gated ion channels [32]. However, ICK peptides with related folds but different sequences often show altered selectivity for ion channels, indicative of promiscuous pharmacophore interactions. δ-Conotoxin TxVIA has been reported to show a prominent hydrophobic patch covering one side of the peptide surface (Figure 6), which was proposed to be crucial for sodium channel binding [33], with our work confirming that TxVIA is non-functional at mammalian Na$_V$s. Interestingly, our docking results reveal that the side opposite to the prominent hydrophobic patch of TxVIA is involved in its binding to DIV extracellular loops of Na$_V$1.7 (Figure 6), suggesting the hydrophobic patch in TxVIA only contributes to Na$_V$ channel affinity. Other Ca$_V$3.x peptide blockers with selectivity for Ca$_V$3.2 include two hydrophobic tarantula toxins PsPTx3 [34,35] and ProTx-II [21] which also inhibits Na$_V$1.7 [20]. Previous structure activity relationship (SAR) studies on ProTx-II reveal that hydrophobic patch interactions with membrane lipids are required for high affinity interactions with hNa$_V$1.7 [36] and Na$_V$1.5 [37]. Ca$_V$3.2 selective peptide blockers also typically show a prominent hydrophobic face, whereas non-hydrophobic peptide blocker ProTx-I inhibits Ca$_V$3.1 [21,25,38]. Indeed, our docking studies suggest that TxVIA also binds to the DIV S3-S4 linker of Ca$_V$3.1 through a more polar surface and not through the adjacent prominent hydrophobic patch (Figure 6).

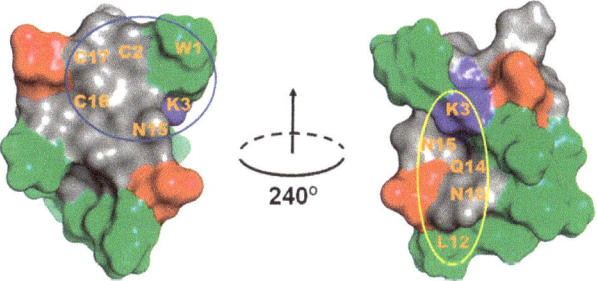

Figure 6. TxVIA (PDB 1FU3) structure pair obtained by 240° horizontal rotation. Peptide surface presented with blue and red colours indicate positive and negative charged residues, respectively, and green colour indicates hydrophobic uncharged residues. The predicted buried surface of TxVIA binding to Na$_V$1.7 is circled in blue and the predicted buried surface of TxVIA binding to Ca$_V$3.1 is circled in yellow. The predicted interacting residues are labelled.

In conclusion, we have identified that δ-conotoxin TxVIA modulates mammalian Ca$_V$3.x, but not mammalian Na$_V$ channels. TxVIA represents a promising new tool to improve our understanding of the molecular mechanism and determinants of activation and inactivation of the different Na$_V$1.x and Ca$_V$3.x subtypes.

4. Materials and Methods

All reagents were used as purchased from Sigma-Aldrich without further purification.

4.1. LC/MS Analysis of TxVIA Distribution in the C. textile Venom Duct

Thirteen adult *C. textile* specimens collected from One Tree Island on the Great Barrier Reef (Queensland, Australia) were sacrificed and dissected into four sections on ice. The crude venom was extracted into 30% acetonitrile, acidified with 0.1 formic acid. The collected 52 crude *C. textile* samples from each of the four duct sections (5 µL) were chromatographically separated on an ultra HPLC system (Shimadzu Scientific, Rydalmere, Australia) directly coupled to a 5600 TripleTOF MS (SCIEX, Foster City, USA). The LC separation was achieved using a Zorbax C_{18} 4.6 × 150 mm column at a linear 1.3% B (acetonitrile/0.1% formic acid (aq)) min^{-1} gradient with a flow rate of 0.2 ml min^{-1} over 90 min. Data were acquired over a time-of-flight (TOF) mass range of 350–2200 Da with an ion spray voltage of 5500 V (CUR 25, TEM 500, GS1 50 and GS2 60). Acquired data were then analysed with Sciex Analyst^{TF} 1.6 software.

4.2. C. textile Crude Venom Fractionation for the Collection of Native TxVIA

Solvent A consists of 0.05% trifluoroacetic acid (TFA) in milli-Q water, whereas solvent B consists of 0.043% TFA and 90% acetonitrile in water. 1.4 mg of lyophilised *C. textile* crude venom dissolved in water with 30% solvent B was loaded using an UltiMate 3000 analytical autosampler (Dionex, Sunnyvale, CA) onto a 00G-4053-E0 *Jupiter*®(Phenomenex, Torrance, CA, USA) 5 µm *C18* 300 Å, 250 × 4.6 mm analytical reversed phase high performance liquid chromatography (RP-HPLC) column and eluted at a flow rate of 0.7 mL/min over 100 min. The elution was monitored at 214 nm.

The following gradient generated by an UltiMate 3000 pump was used to fractionate the *C. textile* crude venom: A constant 5% solvent B over 5 min, 5–80% solvent B over 75 min, 80–90% solvent B over 1 min, a constant 90% solvent B over 4 min, 90–5% solvent B over 1 min, and a constant 5% solvent B over 1 min.

A solvent blank run using the same gradient and equilibration with 5% solvent B for 15 min preceded each separation. Fractions were collected every 1 min over 80 min with a Gilson FC 204 automatic fraction collector (Gilson, Middleton, WI). Collected fractions were transferred into 1.5 mL Eppendorf tubes, dried in a speed vacuum concentrator, resuspended in 100 µL of milli-Q water, vortexed and stored at −20 °C prior to assaying. Peptide concentrations were measured using the NanoDrop One (Thermo Scientific, MA, US). All solvents used were HPLC grade.

4.3. MS and MS/MS Analysis and Sequence Determination of Native TxVIA

4.3.1. MALDI-TOF Mass Spectrometry

Venom peptide masses were verified by matrix-assisted laser desorption/ionisation time-of-flight mass spectrometry (MALDI-TOF MS) using the 4700 Proteomics Bioanalyzer (Applied Biosystems, CA, USA). Venom fractions in water obtained from RP-HPLC were mixed with the matrix CHCA (5 mg/mL in 50% ACN, 1% FA) in 1:1 (v/v) ratio and spotted on a MALDI plate. MALDI-TOF spectra were collected in reflector positive mode and the reported masses are monoisotopic M + H$^+$ ions.

4.3.2. Reduction and Alkylation of Cysteine Residues

45 µL peptide solution was reduced and alkylated with 50 µL of reduction/alkylation cocktail (containing 97.5% acetonitrile, 2% iodoethanol, and 0.5% triethylphosphine by volume) in 50 mM ammonium carbonate solution (pH 11), capped and incubated at 37 °C for 2 h. The sample was then uncapped and evaporated on a speed vacuum for more than 1 h. Dried samples were kept in −80 °C before use.

4.3.3. Trypsin Digestion

Reduced and alkylated peptide was reconstituted with 20 µL of 50 mM ammonium bicarbonate solution (pH 8). Peptide digestion was achieved in 40 ng/µL modified sequencing grade trypsin (Promega, Madison, WI, USA) incubated at 37 °C overnight. Digestion was terminated by adding 5 µL of 5% formic acid.

4.3.4. LC-MS/MS Analysis and Sequence Determination of Native TxVIA

The tryptic peptides (15 µL) were analysed with chromatographic separation using an ultra HPLC system (Shimadzu Scientific, Rydalmere, Australia) directly coupled to a 5600 TripleTOF MS (SCIEX, Foster City, USA). Data were acquired for 55 min 2 s with an ion spray voltage of 5500 V (CUR 25, TEM 500, GS1 50 and GS2 60). ProteinPilot™ 4.0 software (SCIEX) with the Paragon Algorithm was used for protein identification. Tandem mass spectrometry (MS/MS) data was searched against database of *C. textile* from conoserver (http://conoserver.org/). The search parameters were defined as iodoethanol modified for cysteine alkylation and trypsin as the digestion enzyme.

4.4. Cell Culture and Transient Expression

The human embryonic kidney 293 (HEK293) cell line expressing human $Ca_V3.2$ or $Ca_V3.3$ (kind gift from Emmanuel Bourinet, University of Montpellier, France) were cultured under 5% carbon dioxide at 37 °C in Dulbecco's modified Eagle's medium (DMEM), Glutamax (Gibco, Life Technologies, Carlsbad, CA, US) supplemented with 10% (v/v) fetal bovine serum (FBS), 100 U/mL penicillin, 100 µg/mL streptomycin (Gibco, Life Technologies) and 750 µg/mL geneticin (G418) (Gibco, Life Technologies). The Chinese hamster ovary (CHO) cell lines (Emmanuel Bourinet, Montpellier, France) expressing human $Ca_V3.1$ were cultured under 5% carbon dioxide at 37 °C in Minimum Essential Medium Eagle-alpha modification (α-MEM) Glutamax (Gibco, Life Technologies), supplemented with 10% (v/v) FBS and 300 µg/mL geneticin (G418) (Gibco, Life Technologies). The human neuroblastoma SH-SY5Y cells (Victor Diaz, Goettingen, Germany) were cultured under 5% carbon dioxide at 37 °C in RPMI 1640 antibiotic-free medium (Invitrogen, Carlsbad, CA, US), supplemented with 15% FBS and 2 mM GlutaMAX™ (Invitrogen). Dulbecco's phosphate-buffered saline (DPBS) (Gibco, Life Technologies) was used to wash the cells, and 0.25% Trypsin-EDTA (Gibco, Life Technologies) was used to detach cells from the flask surface. They were split in a ratio of 1:5 (ideally 10,000 cells/cm^2) when they reached 70–80% confluency (every 2–3 days). Transiently transfected $Na_V1.7$ HEK293T cells were used in the sodium channel FLIPR assay. HEK293T cells were cultured under 5% carbon dioxide at 37 °C in DMEM Glutamax supplemented with 10% (v/v) FBS. DPBS was used to wash the cells, and 0.25% Trypsin-EDTA was used to detach cells from the flask surface. The cells were split and seeded at 3 million cells per T75 flask, to reach 70–80% confluency after 24 h. The next day, 10 µg plasmid DNA of mouse $Na_V1.7$ α subunit (GenScript, Piscataway, USA) was incubated in 500 µL serum-free DMEM Glutamax with 30 µL FuGENE HD transfection reagent (Promega Corporation, Madison, WI, USA) (1:3 DNA/Fugene ratio) for 20 min, and then the mixture was added into the cell flask slowly, drop by drop. After the transfection, the cells were cultured under 5% carbon dioxide at 37 °C for 16 h and then moved to a 28 °C incubator prior to use.

4.5. Sodium Channel FLIPR Assay

SH-SY5Y cells or transiently transfected $Na_V1.7$ HEK293T cells were seeded into 384-well black wall clear bottom plates at a density of 15,000 cells or 30,000 cells per well, respectively, resulting in 90–95% confluency after 24 h. The media were then removed from the wells and replaced with 20 µL of 10% red membrane potential dye (Molecular Devices, Sunnyvale, CA) in physiological salt solution (PSS) containing 5.9 mM KCl, 1.4 mM $MgCl_2$, 10 mM HEPES, 1.2 mM NaH_2PO_4, 5 mM $NaHCO_3$, 140 mM NaCl, 11.5 mM glucose, 1.8 mM $CaCl_2$ and 0.1% BSA at pH 7.4. The cells were incubated for 30 min at 37 °C in the presence of 5% carbon dioxide. The plates were placed in the FLIPR^{TETRA} (Molecular Devices, Sunnyvale, CA, USA) programmed to record the fluorescence responses under baseline fluorescence 1500–2000 arbitrary fluorescence units (AFU), emission wavelength 565–625 nm, and excitation wavelength 510–545 nm. Prior to the addition of PSS (0.1% BSA) with or without peptide or 10 µM/1 µM TTX, five baseline fluorescence readings were recorded. The fluorescence readings were then recorded once every two seconds over a period of 600 s, resulting in a total of 305 reads before the agonist was added. One fluorescence reading was taken before the second addition.

After PSS (0.1% BSA) for negative control or agonist containing 40–50 μM veratridine was loaded, the fluorescence readings were recorded every two seconds for 600 s, resulting in a total 301 reads. *n* independent experiments were conducted in triplicates. Raw fluorescence readings in the form of relative light units were converted to response over baseline using ScreenWorks®(Molecular Devices, version 3.2.0.14) software.

4.6. T-type Calcium Channel Window Current FLIPR Assays

HEK293 cells stably expressing $Ca_V3.2$ were seeded into 384-well black wall clear bottom plates (Corning, Lowell, MA, US) at a density of 30,000 cells per well. Once the cells reached 80–90% confluency after 24 h, the media were removed from the wells and replaced with 20 μL of 10% calcium 4 dye (Molecular Devices, Sunnyvale, CA, USA) in Hank's balanced salt solution-HEPES (HBSS-HEPES) (containing 5 mM KCl, 10 mM HEPES, 140 mM NaCl, 10 mM glucose and 0.5 mM $CaCl_2$, pH 7.4) with 0.1% bovine serum albumin (BSA). The cells were incubated for 30 min at 37 °C in the presence of 5% carbon dioxide. The plates were placed in the FLIPR^{TETRA} programmed to measure maximum fluorescence intensity following a second addition of the agonist 5 mM $CaCl_2$. The data acquisition parameters were adjusted as follows: baseline fluorescence 1500–2000 AFU, emission wavelength 515–575 nm, excitation wavelength 470–495 nm. Prior to the addition of HBSS-HEPES (0.1% BSA) with or without peptide, five baseline fluorescence readings were recorded. The fluorescence readings were then recorded once every two seconds over a period of 600 s, resulting in a total of 305 reads before the agonist was added. One fluorescence reading was taken before the second addition. After $CaCl_2$ was loaded, the fluorescence readings were recorded every second for 300 s, resulting in a total 301 reads. Raw fluorescence readings in the form of relative light units were converted to response over baseline using ScreenWorks®(Molecular Devices, version 3.2.0.14) software [15].

4.7. Whole-Cell Patch-Clamp Electrophysiology

Whole-cell patch-clamp experiments were performed on an automated electrophysiology platform QPatch 16 X (Sophion Bioscience A/S, Ballerup, Denmark) in single-hole configuration using 16-channel planar patch chip QPlates (Sophion Bioscience A/S). The extracellular recording solution contained: 157 mM TEACl, 0.5 mM $MgCl_2$, 5 mM $CaCl_2$ and 10 mM HEPES; pH 7.4 adjusted with TEAOH; and osmolarity 320 mOsm. The intracellular pipette solution contained: 140 mM CsF, 1 mM EGTA, 10 mM HEPES and 10 mM NaCl; pH 7.2 adjusted with CsOH; and osmolarity 325 mOsm. TxVIA was diluted in extracellular recording solution with 0.1% BSA at the concentrations stated, and the TxVIA effects were compared to the control (extracellular solution with 0.1% BSA) parameters within the same cell. TxVIA incubation time varied from two (for the highest concentration) to five (for the lowest concentration) minutes by applying the voltage protocol 10–30 times at 10 s intervals to ensure steady-state inhibition was achieved. The effects of TxVIA were obtained using 200 ms voltage steps to peak potential from a holding potential of −90 mV. Current–voltage (I–V) relationships were obtained by holding the cells at a potential of −100 mV before applying 50 ms pulses to potentials from −75 to +50 mV every 5 s in 5 mV increments. Data were fitted with a single Boltzmann distribution: $I/I_{max} = (1 + \exp(V − V_{50})/k)^{-1}$, where V_{50} is the half-availability voltage and k is the slope factor. A single-voltage protocol was applied in between to measure the TxVIA effect. One cell was considered as an independent experiment. Off-line data analysis was performed using QPatch Assay Software v5.6 (Sophion Bioscience A/S) and Excel 2013 (Microsoft Corporation, Redmond, WA, USA).

4.8. Homology Modeling and Molecular Docking

Homology models of human $Ca_V3.2$ and $Ca_V3.3$ were generated by SWISS-MODEL [39] using human $Ca_V3.1$ Cryo-EM structure [24] as template. FASTA sequences for human $Ca_V3.2$ and $Ca_V3.3$ were obtained from UniProt and used as query sequences. The resulting models were energy minimised using the GROMOS force field, validated by Ramachandran plot analysis, visualised in PyMol and used for molecular docking using Autodock Vina [40]. For molecular docking of TxVIA in human $Na_V1.7$, we used the DIV S3-S4 linker of previously published human Na$_V$1.7-β1-β2 Cryo-EM structure (PDB 6J8I) [19], as well as the DII S3-S4 linker (missing in the structure of 6J8I) of human Na$_V$1.7 Cryo-EM structure (PDB 6N4I) [23]. To define the search space for the DIV S3-S4 linker of the hNa$_V$1.7 structure, a grid box with the following dimensions: center x = 96.256, center y = 136.521, center z = 155.042 was used. To define the search space for the DII S3-S4 linker of hNa$_V$1.7 structure, a grid box with the following dimensions: center x = 82.85, center y = 288.228, center z = 213.878, was used. The size of the grid box for all the docking in hNa$_V$1.7 was as follows: size x = 30, size y = 30, size z = 30. For molecular docking of hCa$_V$3.1, hCa$_V$3.2, hCa$_V$3.3 DIV S3-S4 linker with TxVIA, a grid box with the following dimensions: center x = 166.339, center y = 123.395, center z = 199.419 was used. The size of the grid box for all the docking in hCa$_V$3.x was as follows: size x = 25, size y = 25, size z = 25. The exhaustiveness for the search was set to 8.

4.9. Evaluation of Zebrafish Pain Behaviours after Intramuscular Injection of TxVIA

Zebrafish were maintained using standard husbandry procedures, conforming to ethical guidelines of the animal ethics committees at the University of Queensland. Six-month old male zebrafish with similar body size and weight were prepared for the assay. Samples were tested via intramuscular injections (5 µL) using a Hamilton syringe (Sigma-Aldrich no. 20795-U). Different concentrations of TxVIA were injected intramuscularly, and the same volume of saline sterilised water was used as control. Three fish were injected per condition. Injected animals were placed in 500 mL containers and their swimming tracks/behaviours were recorded using a custom Zebrabox revolution (Viewpoint) imaging platform and as previously described [41,42]. The animals were observed using the automatic imaging platform for 15 min in dark condition followed by manual monitoring in laboratory light conditions at 28 °C for up to 24 h post-injections. Bursts of erratic swimming were recorded as an indicator of pain behaviours as previously described [14,43].

4.10. Data Analysis

Data were plotted and analysed using GraphPad Prism v8.2.1 (GraphPad Software Inc., San Diego, CA, USA). A four-parameter logistic Hill equation with variable Hill coefficients was fitted to the data for concentration-response curves. Data are means ± SEM of n independent experiments. Statistical analysis was performed with a paired Student's t-test with statistical significance at $p < 0.05$.

Author Contributions: Conceptualisation, R.J.L.; methodology, D.W., S.W.A.H., J.G., M.M.H. and L.R.; validation, D.W., S.W.A.H., J.G., M.M.H., F.C.C., L.R. and R.J.L.; formal analysis, D.W., M.M.H., S.W.A.H. and J.G.; sample preparation, D.W. and S.W.A.H.; calcium channel activity investigation, D.W.; sodium channel activity investigation, D.W. and M.M.H.; homology modeling and molecular docking, M.M.H. and D.W.; zebrafish behavioural investigation, D.W. and J.G.; data Curation, D.W.; writing—original draft preparation, D.W.; writing—review and editing, D.W., S.W.A.H., J.G., M.M.H., F.C.C., L.R. and R.J.L.; supervision, L.R. and R.J.L.; funding acquisition, R.J.L. All authors have read and agreed to the published version of the manuscript.

Funding: This research was supported by NHMRC Program Grant number APP1072113 and an NHMRC Principal Research Fellowship (to RJL). The zebrafish component has also been supported by a NHMRC Investigator Grant APP1174145 and a Rebecca L. Cooper Medical research Project Grant PG2019405 (to JG).

Acknowledgments: The authors thank Emmanuel Bourinet for donating stable cell lines for T-type calcium channels, Alun Jones for helping with mass spectrometric analysis and all the Lewis group members who have contributed to the *C. textile* maintenance and venom collection.

Conflicts of Interest: The authors declare no conflict of interest.

References

1. Hillyard, D.R.; Olivera, B.M.; Woodward, S.; Corpuz, G.P.; Gray, W.R.; Ramilo, C.A.; Cruz, L.J. A molluskivorous Conus toxin: Conserved frameworks in conotoxins. *Biochemistry* **1989**, *28*, 358–361. [CrossRef]
2. Fainzilber, M.; Gordon, D.; Hasson, A.; Spira, M.E.; Zlotkin, E. Mollusc-specific toxins from the venom of Conus textile neovicarius. *Eur. J. Biochem.* **1991**, *202*, 589–595. [CrossRef]

3. Hasson, A.; Fainzilber, M.; Gordon, D.; Zlotkin, E.; Spira, M.E. Alteration of sodium currents by new peptide toxins from the venom of a molluscivorous Conus snail. *Eur. J. Neurosci.* **1993**, *5*, 56–64. [CrossRef] [PubMed]

4. Fainzilber, M.; Kofman, O.; Zlotkin, E.; Gordon, D. A new neurotoxin receptor site on sodium channels is identified by a conotoxin that affects sodium channel inactivation in molluscs and acts as an antagonist in rat brain. *J. Biol. Chem.* **1994**, *269*, 2574–2580. [PubMed]

5. Gonoi, T.; Ashida, K.; Feller, D.; Schmidt, J.; Fujiwara, M.; Catterall, W.A. Mechanism of action of a polypeptide neurotoxin from the coral Goniopora on sodium channels in mouse neuroblastoma cells. *Mol. Pharmacol.* **1986**, *29*, 347. [PubMed]

6. Gonoi, T.; Ohizumi, Y.; Kobayashi, J.; Nakamura, H.; Catterall, W.A. Actions of a polypeptide toxin from the marine snail Conus striatus on voltage-sensitive sodium channels. *Mol. Pharmacol.* **1987**, *32*, 691–698.

7. Kostyuk, P.; Mironov, S.; Shuba, Y.M. Two ion-selecting filters in the calcium channel of the somatic membrane of mollusc neurons. *J. Membr. Biol.* **1983**, *76*, 83–93. [CrossRef]

8. Spafford, J.D.; Spencer, A.N.; Gallin, W.J. Genomic organization of a voltage-gated Na$^+$ channel in a hydrozoan jellyfish: Insights into the evolution of voltage-gated Na$^+$ channel genes. *Recept. Channels* **1999**, *6*, 493–506.

9. Gray, L.S.; Macdonald, T.L. The pharmacology and regulation of T type calcium channels: New opportunities for unique therapeutics for cancer. *Cell Calcium* **2006**, *40*, 115–120. [CrossRef]

10. Rossier, M.F. T-type calcium channel: A privileged gate for calcium entry and control of adrenal steroidogenesis. *Front. Endocrinol.* **2016**, *7*, 43. [CrossRef] [PubMed]

11. Wang, D.; Ragnarsson, L.; Lewis, R.J. T type calcium channels in health and disease. *Curr. Med. Chem.* **2020**, *27*, 3098–3122. [CrossRef]

12. Vetter, I.; Mozar, C.A.; Durek, T.; Wingerd, J.S.; Alewood, P.F.; Christie, M.J.; Lewis, R.J. Characterisation of Na$_V$ types endogenously expressed in human SH-SY5Y neuroblastoma cells. *Biochem. Pharmacol.* **2012**, *83*, 1562–1571. [CrossRef] [PubMed]

13. Khan, K.M.; Collier, A.D.; Meshalkina, D.A.; Kysil, E.V.; Khatsko, S.L.; Kolesnikova, T.; Morzherin, Y.Y.; Warnick, J.E.; Kalueff, A.V.; Echevarria, D.J. Zebrafish models in neuropsychopharmacology and CNS drug discovery. *Br. J. Pharmacol.* **2017**, *174*, 1925–1944. [CrossRef] [PubMed]

14. Speedie, N.; Gerlai, R. Alarm substance induced behavioral responses in zebrafish (*Danio rerio*). *Behav. Brain Res.* **2008**, *188*, 168–177. [CrossRef] [PubMed]

15. Wang, D.; Neupane, P.; Ragnarsson, L.; Capon, R.J.; Lewis, R.J. Synthesis of pseudellone analogs and characterization as novel T-type calcium channel blockers. *Mar. Drugs* **2018**, *16*, 475. [CrossRef]

16. Thomsen, W.J.; Catterall, W.A. Localization of the receptor site for α-scorpion toxins by antibody mapping: Implications for sodium channel topology. *Proc. Natl. Acad. Sci. USA* **1989**, *86*, 10161–10165. [CrossRef]

17. Rogers, J.C.; Qu, Y.; Tanada, T.N.; Scheuer, T.; Catterall, W.A. Molecular determinants of high affinity binding of α-scorpion toxin and sea anemone toxin in the S3-S4 extracellular loop in domain IV of the Na$^+$ channel α subunit. *J. Biol. Chem.* **1996**, *271*, 15950–15962. [CrossRef]

18. Clairfeuille, T.; Cloake, A.; Infield, D.T.; Llongueras, J.P.; Arthur, C.P.; Li, Z.R.; Jian, Y.; Martin-Eauclaire, M.-F.; Bougis, P.E.; Ciferri, C. Structural basis of α-scorpion toxin action on Na$_V$ channels. *Science* **2019**, *363*, eaav8573. [CrossRef]

19. Shen, H.; Liu, D.; Wu, K.; Lei, J.; Yan, N. Structures of human Na$_V$1.7 channel in complex with auxiliary subunits and animal toxins. *Science* **2019**, *363*, 1303–1308. [CrossRef]

20. Schmalhofer, W.A.; Calhoun, J.; Burrows, R.; Bailey, T.; Kohler, M.G.; Weinglass, A.B.; Kaczorowski, G.J.; Garcia, M.L.; Koltzenburg, M.; Priest, B.T. ProTx-II, a selective inhibitor of Na$_V$1.7 sodium channels, blocks action potential propagation in nociceptors. *Mol. Pharmacol.* **2008**, *74*, 1476–1484. [CrossRef]

21. Bladen, C.; Hamid, J.; Souza, I.A.; Zamponi, G.W. Block of T-type calcium channels by protoxins I and II. *Mol. Brain* **2014**, *7*, 36. [CrossRef] [PubMed]

22. Stevens, M.; Peigneur, S.; Tytgat, J. Neurotoxins and their binding areas on voltage-gated sodium channels. *Front. Pharmacol.* **2011**, *2*, 71. [CrossRef] [PubMed]

23. Xu, H.; Li, T.; Rohou, A.; Arthur, C.P.; Tzakoniati, F.; Wong, E.; Estevez, A.; Kugel, C.; Franke, Y.; Chen, J.; et al. Structural basis of Na$_V$1.7 inhibition by a gating-modifier spider toxin. *Cell* **2019**, *176*, 702–715. [CrossRef]

24. Zhao, Y.; Huang, G.; Wu, Q.; Wu, K.; Li, R.; Lei, J.; Pan, X.; Yan, N. Cryo-EM structures of apo and antagonist-bound human Ca$_V$3.1. *Nature* **2019**, *576*, 492–497. [CrossRef] [PubMed]

25. Ohkubo, T.; Yamazaki, J.; Kitamura, K. Tarantula toxin ProTx-I differentiates between human T-type voltage-gated Ca^{2+} Channels $Ca_V3.1$ and $Ca_V3.2$. *J. Pharmacol. Sci.* **2010**, *112*, 452–458. [CrossRef] [PubMed]

26. Uebele, V.N.; Nuss, C.E.; Fox, S.V.; Garson, S.L.; Cristescu, R.; Doran, S.M.; Kraus, R.L.; Santarelli, V.P.; Li, Y.; Barrow, J.C. Positive allosteric interaction of structurally diverse T-type calcium channel antagonists. *Cell Biochem. Biophys.* **2009**, *55*, 81–93. [CrossRef] [PubMed]

27. Tringham, E.; Powell, K.L.; Cain, S.M.; Kuplast, K.; Mezeyova, J.; Weerapura, M.; Eduljee, C.; Jiang, X.; Smith, P.; Morrison, J.-L. T-type calcium channel blockers that attenuate thalamic burst firing and suppress absence seizures. *Sci. Transl. Med.* **2012**, *4*, 121ra19. [CrossRef]

28. Bourinet, E.; Alloui, A.; Monteil, A.; Barrere, C.; Couette, B.; Poirot, O.; Pages, A.; McRory, J.; Snutch, T.P.; Eschalier, A. Silencing of the $Ca_V3.2$ T-type calcium channel gene in sensory neurons demonstrates its major role in nociception. *EMBO J.* **2005**, *24*, 315–324. [CrossRef]

29. Maeda, Y.; Aoki, Y.; Sekiguchi, F.; Matsunami, M.; Takahashi, T.; Nishikawa, H.; Kawabata, A. Hyperalgesia induced by spinal and peripheral hydrogen sulfide: Evidence for involvement of $Ca_V3.2$ T-type calcium channels. *Pain* **2009**, *142*, 127–132. [CrossRef]

30. Choi, S.; Na, H.; Kim, J.; Lee, J.; Lee, S.; Kim, D.; Park, J.; Chen, C.C.; Campbell, K.; Shin, H.S. Attenuated pain responses in mice lacking $Ca_V3.2$ T-type channels. *Genes Brain Behav.* **2007**, *6*, 425–431. [CrossRef]

31. Dutertre, S.; Jin, A.-H.; Vetter, I.; Hamilton, B.; Sunagar, K.; Lavergne, V.; Dutertre, V.; Fry, B.G.; Antunes, A.; Venter, D.J. Evolution of separate predation-and defence-evoked venoms in carnivorous cone snails. *Nat. Commun.* **2014**, *5*, 3521. [CrossRef] [PubMed]

32. Craik, D.J.; Daly, N.L.; Waine, C. The cystine knot motif in toxins and implications for drug design. *Toxicon* **2001**, *39*, 43–60. [CrossRef]

33. Kohno, T.; Sasaki, T.; Kobayashi, K.; Fainzilber, M.; Sato, K. Three-dimensional solution structure of the sodium channel agonist/antagonist δ-conotoxin TxVIA. *J. Biol. Chem.* **2002**, *277*, 36387–36391. [CrossRef]

34. Bourinet, E.; Escoubas, P.; Marger, F.; Nargeot, J.; Lazdunski, M. Identification of novel antagonist toxins of T-Type calcium channel for analgesic purposes. U.S. Patent 8,664,179, 4 March 2014.

35. Bourinet, E.; Zamponi, G.W. Block of voltage-gated calcium channels by peptide toxins. *Neuropharmacology* **2017**, *127*, 109–115. [CrossRef] [PubMed]

36. Henriques, S.T.; Deplazes, E.; Lawrence, N.; Cheneval, O.; Chaousis, S.; Inserra, M.; Thongyoo, P.; King, G.F.; Mark, A.E.; Vetter, I. Interaction of tarantula venom peptide ProTx-II with lipid membranes is a prerequisite for its inhibition of human voltage-gated sodium channel $Na_V1.7$. *J. Biol. Chem.* **2016**, *291*, 17049–17065. [CrossRef] [PubMed]

37. Smith, J.J.; Cummins, T.R.; Alphy, S.; Blumenthal, K.M. Molecular interactions of the gating modifier toxin, ProTx-II, with $Na_V1.5$. Implied existence of a novel toxin binding site coupled to activation. *J. Biol. Chem.* **2007**, *282*, 12687–12697. [CrossRef]

38. Priest, B.T.; Blumenthal, K.M.; Smith, J.J.; Warren, V.A.; Smith, M.M. ProTx-I and ProTx-II: Gating modifiers of voltage-gated sodium channels. *Toxicon* **2007**, *49*, 194–201. [CrossRef]

39. Waterhouse, A.; Bertoni, M.; Bienert, S.; Studer, G.; Tauriello, G.; Gumienny, R.; Heer, F.T.; de Beer, T.A.P.; Rempfer, C.; Bordoli, L.; et al. SWISS-MODEL: Homology modelling of protein structures and complexes. *Nucleic Acids Res.* **2018**, *46*, W296–W303. [CrossRef]

40. Trott, O.; Olson, A.J. AutoDock Vina: Improving the speed and accuracy of docking with a new scoring function, efficient optimization, and multithreading. *J. Comput. Chem.* **2010**, *31*, 455–461. [CrossRef]

41. Giacomotto, J.; Rinkwitz, S.; Becker, T.S. Effective heritable gene knockdown in zebrafish using synthetic microRNAs. *Nat. Commun.* **2015**, *6*, 1–11. [CrossRef]

42. Laird, A.S.; Mackovski, N.; Rinkwitz, S.; Becker, T.S.; Giacomotto, J. Tissue-specific models of spinal muscular atrophy confirm a critical role of SMN in motor neurons from embryonic to adult stages. *Hum. Mol. Genet.* **2016**, *25*, 1728–1738. [CrossRef] [PubMed]

43. Himaya, S.W.A.; Jin, A.-H.; Dutertre, S.; Giacomotto, J.; Mohialdeen, H.; Vetter, I.; Alewood, P.F.; Lewis, R.J. Comparative venomics reveals the complex prey capture strategy of the piscivorous cone snail *Conus catus*. *J. Proteome Res* **2015**, *14*, 4372–4381. [CrossRef] [PubMed]

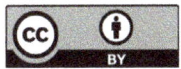

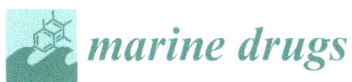

Article

RgIA4 Accelerates Recovery from Paclitaxel-Induced Neuropathic Pain in Rats

Peter N. Huynh [1,*,‡], **Denise Giuvelis** [2,†], **Sean Christensen** [1,†], **Kerry L. Tucker** [2,3] and **J. Michael McIntosh** [1,4,5]

1   School of Biological Sciences, University of Utah, Salt Lake City, UT 84112, USA
2   Center for Excellence in the Neurosciences, University of New England, Biddeford, ME 04005, USA
3   Dept. of Biomedical Sciences, College of Osteopathic Medicine, University of New England, Biddeford, ME 04005, USA
4   George E. Whalen Veterans Affairs Medical Center, Salt Lake City, UT 84112, USA
5   Department of Psychiatry, University of Utah, Salt Lake City, UT 84112, USA
*   Correspondence: Peter.Huynh@utah.edu; Tel.: +1-801-581-8370
†   These authors contributed equally to this work.
‡   Current address: 257 S 1400 E Room 201, Salt Lake City, UT 84112, USA.

Received: 27 November 2019; Accepted: 18 December 2019; Published: 21 December 2019

Abstract: Chemotherapeutic drugs are widely utilized in the treatment of human cancers. Painful chemotherapy-induced neuropathy is a common, debilitating, and dose-limiting side effect for which there is currently no effective treatment. Previous studies have demonstrated the potential utility of peptides from the marine snail from the genus *Conus* for the treatment of neuropathic pain. α-Conotoxin RgIA and a potent analog, RgIA4, have previously been shown to prevent the development of neuropathy resulting from the administration of oxaliplatin, a platinum-based antineoplastic drug. Here, we have examined its efficacy against paclitaxel, a chemotherapeutic drug that works by a mechanism of action distinct from that of oxaliplatin. Paclitaxel was administered at 2 mg/kg (intraperitoneally (IP)) every other day for a total of 8 mg/kg. Sprague Dawley rats that were co-administered RgIA4 at 80 µg/kg (subcutaneously (SC)) once daily, five times per week, for three weeks showed significant recovery from mechanical allodynia by day 31. Notably, the therapeutic effects reached significance 12 days after the last administration of RgIA4, which is suggestive of a rescue mechanism. These findings support the effects of RgIA4 in multiple chemotherapeutic models and the investigation of α9α10 nicotinic acetylcholine receptors (nAChRs) as a non-opioid target in the treatment of chronic pain.

Keywords: nicotinic; chemotherapy; paclitaxel; taxane; neuropathic pain; α9α10; conotoxin

1. Introduction

Neuropathic pain is a type of chronic pain that stems from the damage or disease of the sensory nervous system that affects an estimated 6.9–10% of the general population [1]. This type of pathological pain has many causes, including traumatic nerve injury, metabolic disorders such as diabetes, and chemical damage from chemotherapeutics [2]. Paclitaxel (Figure 1) is an anti-cancer drug of the taxane family, initially extracted from the bark of the Pacific yew (*Taxus brevifolia*), and perhaps the most well-known natural-product chemotherapeutic. It is used as a first-line treatment for breast, ovarian, and non-small cell lung cancers [3]. Several chemotherapies from different drug families, including taxane- and platinum-based drugs, have been characterized to produce painful neuropathies as a side effect. In the context of cancer therapies, these side effects can be more than disruptive as they are often dose-limiting in treatment regimens [4].

Patients have exhibited several types of neuropathies, including numbness, chronic pain, and allodynia (painful hypersensitivity) to mechanical or thermal stimuli [5]. Amongst patients, however, the type, duration, and severity of neuropathy can vary [6]. While the prevalence and manifestations of paclitaxel-induced neuropathy have been well documented, the underlying mechanisms are still being characterized. Several adjuvant treatments have been used in an attempt to combat the effects of chemotherapy-induced peripheral neuropathy (CIPN). However, there are currently no FDA-approved medications for the prevention or treatment of CIPN.

Cone snails have historically displayed a repertoire of therapeutic molecules. The venomous marine gastropods of the genus *Conus* are a diverse collection of snails that have developed complex hunting and envenomation strategies. The venoms of these snails contain hundreds of unique peptides, and the contents of these venoms can also change in response to defensive or predatory stimuli [7]. Cone snails have refined a suite of bioactive peptides that can exquisitely and potently discriminate among receptors involved in neurotransmission. These targets include G-protein-coupled receptors and voltage- and ligand-gated ion channels [8]. The chemical arsenal of each snail also contains bioactive compounds that have been characterized as prey-endogenous mimetics, such as the insulin-like peptide used by *Conus geographus*, which more closely resembles fish insulin than its own [9]. The discovery of this molecular mimicry strategy spurred the characterization of several other hormone/neuropeptide-like peptides in the venom repertoire of these snails [10].

Currently, there are an estimated 750+ species of cone snails whose venom components include small, disulfide-rich peptides that have been classified into at least 28 different superfamilies. These superfamilies are primarily subdivided by their conserved cysteine frameworks. Further characterization of cone snail venom ducts have also revealed the presence of small molecules that contribute to their venom activity [11]. Previous estimates of 50–200 unique compounds per venom have been expanded nearly 10-fold with the advancement of mass spectroscopy and venomics techniques. These estimates yield a collection of greater than 1 million potential lead peptide compounds to be characterized, less than 1% of which (~10,000) have been partially characterized [12,13]. While advancements in genomics, proteomics, and transcriptomics have rapidly accelerated the discovery of conotoxin peptides, the structural and pharmacological characterization has been rate-limiting. Notably, the ω-conotoxin MVIIA (Prialt®(ziconotide)), a non-opioid drug for intractable pain, remains the only FDA-approved conotoxin-based drug to date [14,15]. The majority of bioactive wealth from cone snail venoms awaits to be characterized. The classification and therapeutic applications of conotoxins have been reviewed in considerable detail [7,8,10,12,14–20].

Among the smallest of the peptides found in *Conus* venoms are the α-conotoxins, which competitively inhibit nicotinic acetylcholine receptors (nAChRs) [16]. α-conotoxins are typically 13–20 amino acids in length and disulfide-constrained. nAChRs are pentamers typically assembled from α and non-α subunits including α1–α10, β1–β4, and γ, δ, and ε in coordinated distributions. There are also homomeric assemblies consisting only of α-subunits. Together, these subunit combinations yield a large diversity of potential nAChR subtypes.

Previously, we have reported the specific block of α9α10 nAChRs by the α-conotoxin RgIA [21,22]. This 13-amino-acid peptide, isolated from the worm-hunting snail *Conus regius*, blocked the rodent α9α10 nAChR with high potency; however, it was found to be approximately 300-fold less potent on the human receptor due to a single amino-acid substitution in the α9 nAChR subunit [23]. The second-generation synthetic analog, RgIA4, was engineered to close this affinity gap across the rodent and human α9α10 nAChRs (IC$_{50}$ rat = 0.9 nM; IC$_{50}$ human = 1.5 nM), and has also been shown to effectively prevent oxaliplatin-induced pain in rats and mice [24,25]. These findings are consistent with previous behavioral and cellular studies that demonstrate native RgIA can prevent the development and/or progression of neuropathic pain in chronic constriction injury and oxaliplatin-induced injury [26–28]. RgIA and several other α-conotoxins from worm-hunting *Conus* species act on ancestral nAChRs such as α9, α10, or α7-containing subtypes. While these α-conotoxins may incapacitate their native prey, their effect on higher-order species is more nuanced, since the target receptors may play roles outside the neuromuscular junction [29]. Here, we show that, in addition to preventing oxaliplatin-derived neuropathic pain, RgIA4 is efficacious in accelerating recovery from paclitaxel-induced neuropathic pain in rats.

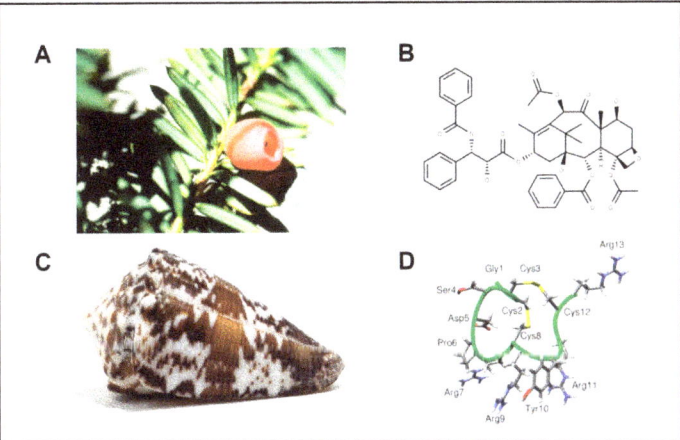

Figure 1. Natural sources of potential therapeutics. (**A**) The needles and berries of a Pacific yew, characteristic of the tree from which paclitaxel was originally extracted. (**B**) Chemical structure of paclitaxel. (**C**) Shell of the worm-hunting snail, *Conus regius*, from which RgIA was originally characterized. (**D**) Structure of the short 13-amino-acid peptide RgIA isolated from *Conus regius*. Image sources: (**A**) Yew Needles and Berries, National Cancer Institute Visuals Online, no. AV-9100-3761. (**C**) *Conus regius* photograph by Peter Huynh.

2. Results

2.1. RgIA4 Accelerates Recovery from Paclitaxel-Induced Allodynia in Sprague Dawley Rats

Semisynthetic taxanes, including paclitaxel, are first-line treatments for the most common solid tumors, but taxane induced peripheral neurotoxicity is a frequent dose-limiting side effect. Sprague Dawley (SD) rats are commonly used to model paclitaxel-mediated CIPN due to the consistent induction of mechanical and thermal allodynia and ease of behavioral readouts compared to mice [30–32]. A clinical formulation of paclitaxel was chosen in order to induce a longer-lasting neuropathic pain effect [31]. Adult SD rats were injected four times intraperitoneally (IP) with paclitaxel (2.0 mg/kg) on days 0, 2, 4, and 6, for a total dosage of 8.0 mg/kg. Over the course of the paclitaxel injections and over the next 12 days, rats were also administered daily subcutaneous (SC) injections of RgIA4 at 16 and 80 µg/kg five days per week (days 0–18) (Figure 2A). To assay for mechanoreceptive properties of paclitaxel-induced neuropathic pain, SD rats were tested through hindpaw von Frey analysis.

Compared to vehicle-injected animals, paclitaxel-injected rats showed a robust, painful sensitization to previously non-painful mechanical stimuli by day 9 which persisted through day 44 (Figure 2B). These effects peaked on day 16, where the paclitaxel (PTX)-saline-treated rats exhibited a pain response from the Von Frey filaments, withdrawing or licking their paw at a mean threshold of 6.2 g, compared to the vehicle-saline-treated rats, whose threshold was at a mean force of 14.6 g. Co-administration of RgIA4 (16 or 80 µg/kg; SC) did not produce analgesic effects during the induction of neuropathic pain (days 0–16).

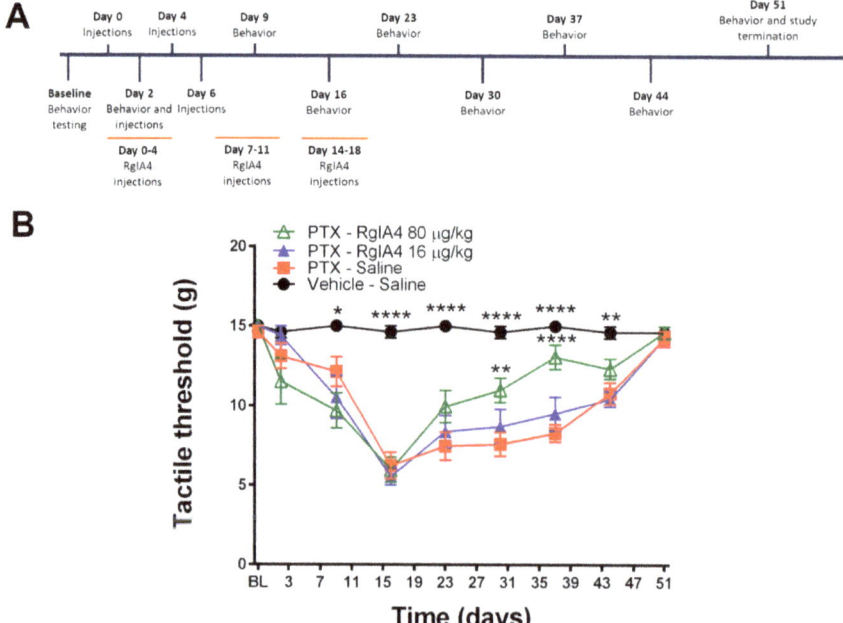

Figure 2. RgIA4 accelerates recovery from mechanical allodynia. (**A**) Study timeline. Sprague Dawley (SD) rats (*n* = 8) were treated with either vehicle (intraperitoneally (IP))-saline (subcutaneously (SC)), 8 mg/kg paclitaxel (PTX) (IP)-saline (SC), 8 mg/kg paclitaxel (IP)-RgIA4 (80 μg/kg; SC), or 8 mg/kg paclitaxel (IP)-RgIA4 (16 μg/kg; SC). Animals were tested for behavior prior to the first dose of paclitaxel (baseline (BL)) and over the course of 51 days. (**B**) Testing results from Von Frey assay. Results are expressed as tactile threshold values in grams (g). Black circles: vehicle-saline; red squares: PTX-saline; blue triangles: PTX-RgIA4 (16 μg/kg); hollow green triangles: PTX-RgIA4 (80 μg/kg). Mean +/- SEM are indicated. Two-way ANOVA was conducted followed by Bonferroni's multiple comparison test, alpha = 0.05. Asterisks denote a significant difference from the PTX-Saline curve (* $p < 0.05$, ** $p < 0.01$, and **** $p < 0.0001$).

By day 23, the paclitaxel-treated groups began a modest recovery from their mechanical allodynia. However, by day 31, rats treated with 80 μg/kg of RgIA4 showed accelerated recovery from the paclitaxel-induced hypersensitivity, reaching significance compared to the paclitaxel-saline-treated rats ($p < 0.01$, as determined by two-way ANOVA followed by Bonferonni's multiple comparison test). The rate of recovery by the RgIA4 (80 μg/kg)-treated rats maximally outpaced all other groups by day 37 ($p < 0.0001$). Remarkably, this therapeutic effect was first reached 12 days after treatment with RgIA4 had been stopped.

Further analysis of thermoreceptive properties revealed no ameliorative effects of RgIA4 at either dosage as determined by a cold plate assay (Figure 3). Neither paclitaxel nor RgIA4 affected heat allodynia, as measured by the Hargreaves test, nor the weight gain of the animals over the course of the experiment (Figure 4). The dosages of 80 and 16 μg/kg were chosen based on previously characterized regimens that effectively produced relief in neuropathic pain models in mice and rats [24,25]. These dosages have been previously reported to produce no adverse effects in motor coordination nor CNS function based on rotarod and Irwin tests [25].

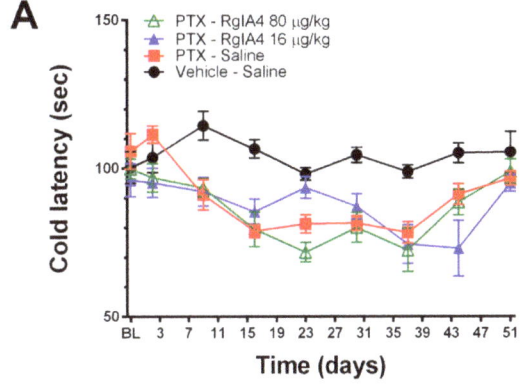

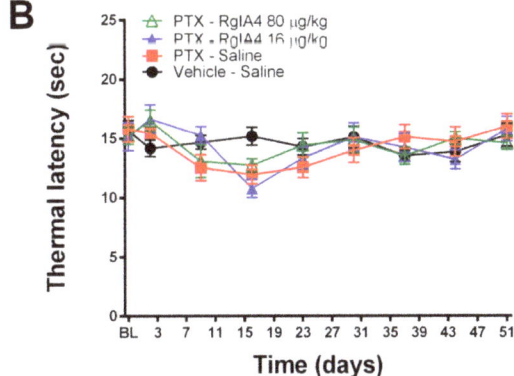

Figure 3. RgIA4 did not reverse cold allodynia and paclitaxel did not induce heat allodynia under these conditions. Testing results from (**A**) cold plate and (**B**) Hargreaves assays following treatment of SD rats (*n* = 8 per group, unless otherwise noted) with a total dose of 8 mg/kg paclitaxel with or without RgIA4 at 80 or 16 µg/kg. Animals were tested for behavior from the first dose of paclitaxel (BL) over the course of 51 days. Results are expressed in (**A**) cold and (**B**) thermal latency times in seconds (s). Black circles: vehicle-saline; red squares: PTX-saline; blue triangles: PTX-RgIA4 (16 µg/kg); hollow green triangles: PTX- RgIA4 (80 µg/kg). Mean +/- SEM are indicated.

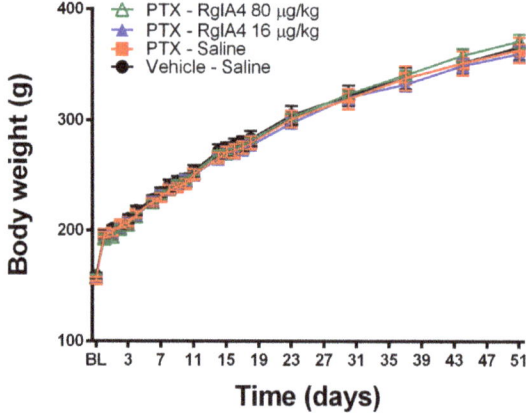

Figure 4. Neither paclitaxel nor RgIA4 significantly affected body weight over time. Changes in rat body weight (in g) are indicated following treatment with a total dose of 8 mg/kg paclitaxel, with or without RgIA4 at 80 or 16 µg/kg. Readings were taken from cohorts of *n* = 8 rats per group, unless otherwise specified. Black circles: vehicle-saline; red squares: PTX-saline; blue triangles: PTX-RgIA4 (16 µg/kg); hollow green triangles: PTX-RgIA4 (80 µg/kg). Mean +/- SEM are indicated.

2.2. Paclitaxel Did Not Induce Mechanical Allodynia in C57BL/6J Mice

Rats have been widely used in models of neuropathic pain. When mice are used, the C57BL/6J mouse is perhaps the most commonly used inbred strain; its entire genome has been sequenced, and a wide variety of transgenics are available. The effectiveness of inducing CIPN pain in C57BL/6J mice with paclitaxel, however, has been reported with varying levels of success. Some previous reports showed robust induction of CIPN by paclitaxel in C57BL/6J mice, while others were not able to create this pain state [32,33]. The diverse genetic background of inbred mouse strains has historically resulted in variable levels of CIPN severity. This has been documented across several strains of mice with both paclitaxel and oxaliplatin as the agent of induction [32,34]. Additional, early genome-wide association studies (GWASs) have suggested genetic predispositions to CIPN pain [35]. This is also reflective of clinical reports, where the severity and duration of painful neuropathy varies between patients [4].

In our experiments, administration of C57BL/6J mice with 2.0 mg/kg of paclitaxel (IP) on days 0, 2, 4, and 6 did not produce a statistically significant change in mechanical allodynia as measured by Von Frey (Supplemental Figure S1). As a measure of neurophysiological integrity, the velocity and amplitudes of sensory nerve action potentials (SNAPs) are commonly used as a readout in both clinical and preclinical settings [36,37]. Previous studies have reported the reduction of action potential amplitude in patients receiving paclitaxel as the duration of their treatment regimen progressed [38]. In our cohort of C57/BL6 mice, there was no change in observed nerve conduction velocities (NCVs) nor amplitudes of SNAPs in the tail between treated and untreated mice (Supplemental Figure S2). Due to the lack of robust induction under these conditions, we did not continue with further behavioral tests in C57BL/6J mice.

3. Discussion

3.1. α9α10 nAChRs as a Target for Pain Treatment

RgIA4 has been previously shown to prevent the induction of CIPN pain by the platinum-based chemotherapeutic, oxaliplatin [24,25]. Since chemotherapeutic agents work by different mechanisms of action to inhibit tumor growth, we wished to assess the activity of RgIA4 in taxane-induced neuropathic pain [39]. Taxanes are effective treatments for breast cancer; however, neuropathic pain is a common side effect. After two years of treatment, over 40% of women indicated that they still experience neuropathy symptoms with compromised long-term quality of life [40,41]. There are currently no recommended agents for the prevention of taxane-induced neuropathic pain. The positive outcome for RgIA4 indicates broader applicability of $\alpha9\alpha10$ nAChR antagonists for preventing symptoms of CIPN.

In this study, the repeated and intermittent administration of clinically-formulated dosages of paclitaxel produced a robust mechanical allodynia which was consistent with previous reports in both humans and rodents [5]. A previously-observed coasting phenomenon was also present in which symptoms could continue and even intensify after cessation of treatment. In this study, symptoms peaked in intensity on day 16, ten days after the last administration of paclitaxel; a similar phenomenon has been reported in clinical settings and successfully reproduced in rodent models [31,42]. The administration of RgIA4 five days per week for three weeks successfully accelerated the recovery from paclitaxel-induced mechanical allodynia in a dose-dependent manner. The effects of RgIA4 only became evident after repeated dosages and did not reach significance until day 30, approximately 12 days after the RgIA4 administration had been discontinued. This delay in efficacy is consistent with our previous reports of both native RgIA in chronic constriction injury models of neuropathic pain and RgIA4 in oxaliplatin-mediated neuropathic pain. The time course of symptom relief is consistent with a disease-modifying effect of RgIA4 rather than just a pain-masking effect [24–26]. In future studies, it will be of interest to assess the effects of RgIA4 that are administered over a longer time frame.

The diversity of cone snails and their venom components have provided a rich pharmaceutical cornucopia of neuroactive compounds. Previously, α-conotoxins such as Vc1.1 and RgIA have been characterized to produce anti-pain effects in rodent models of chronic pain, as have been members of the ω-conotoxin family such as MVIIA [28,43]. MVIIA is commercially available as Prialt®(ziconotide) for the treatment of intractable pain and acts by blocking N-type calcium channels in the CNS. Notably, N-type calcium channels may be inhibited by stimulation of γ-aminobutyric acid type-B (GABA$_B$) receptors or μ-opioid receptors [44–46]. The stimulation of GABA$_B$ receptors has been proposed as the mechanism of action for α-conotoxins Vc1.1 and RgIA [47–52]. We note, however, that the RgIA analog used in the present study, RgIA4, does not have GABA$_B$ or μ–opioid activity [24,25].

It is noteworthy that the analgesic effects of RgIA4 do not become apparent until the discontinuation of treatment. Previous studies of RgIA and RgIA4 have indicated that full analgesic effects may occur after several weeks of treatment [24–26]. This efficacy time course is consistent with a disease-modifying effect that we observed in oxaliplatin-induced neuropathic pain, where RgIA4-treated animals demonstrate anti-allodynic benefits for several weeks after the discontinuation of RgIA4 treatment [24]. This suggests that RgIA4 affects the progression of chronic pain development and recovery, yielding pain relief even after the clearance of RgIA4 from circulation. While neuropathic pain has many different causes, a point of convergence in the progression of disease is neuroinflammation and peripheral nerve damage [2]. $\alpha9\alpha10$ nAChRs have not been shown to be involved in the neurotransmission of pain. However, these receptors have been shown to be expressed in peripheral immune cells and to affect the release of inflammatory cytokines in vitro and the infiltration of immune cells into perineural spaces following chronic constriction injury (CCI) [28,53,54]. While the exact mechanisms by which $\alpha9\alpha10$ nAChR antagonists exert their therapeutic effects have yet to be elucidated, it is likely that the long-term neuroprotective effects are, at least in part, influenced by neuroimmune-mediated mechanisms.

Other $\alpha9\alpha10$ antagonists, structurally unrelated to RgIA4, have also been shown to have analgesic activity in CIPN pain and other neuropathic pain models. Small molecule azaaromatic quaternary ammonium analogs selectively block $\alpha9\alpha10$ nAChRs [55]. The bis-analog, ZZ1-61c, prevented the development of vincristine-induced neuropathic pain [56]. The tetrakis-quaternary ammonium ZZ-204G was analgesic in formalin and CCI models of neuropathic pain [57]. In addition, an entirely different conotoxin peptide, αO-conotoxin GeXIVA, which blocks $\alpha9\alpha10$ nAChRs noncompetitively and lacks GABA$_B$ agonist activity, also reverses oxaliplatin-induced neuropathic pain and CCI pain [58–60].

Conotoxins may be classified by gene superfamily and defined by their signal sequence in the prepropeptide region and their disulfide framework. The α-conotoxins are members of the A-superfamily, which are characterized as two-disulfide-bridged peptides, typically 13–19 amino acids in length, that selectively and competitively inhibit nAChRs [61]. By contrast, αO-conotoxin GeXIVA is from the O1-superfamily, which are three-disulfide-bridged peptides that typically inhibit voltage-gated ion channels [19]. This diverse group of antagonists supports the idea that α9α10 nAChRs are an effective target for reversing and accelerating recovery from neuropathic pain.

3.2. Chemotherapy-Induced Neuropathic Pain and Block of α9α10 nAChRs

Chemotherapeutics of the taxane, vinca-alkaloid, and platinum-based families have different mechanisms of action. Paclitaxel is a member of the taxane family and produces a robust anti-cancer effect by stabilizing microtubule polymers, effectively preventing the disassembly and progression of mitosis [62–64]. Vinca alkaloids also target microtubules, but in a fashion "opposite" to taxanes, do so by destabilizing microtubule formation [65]. By contrast, platinum-based drugs such as oxaliplatin primarily target DNA, creating DNA lesions and adducts, ultimately preventing cell replication [66]. Just as the mechanisms of action between taxanes, vinca alkaloids, and platinum-based drugs are different, the resulting neuropathologies also develop differently. Taxanes cause dysfunction to mitochondria and endoplasmic reticulum calcium signaling as a side effect of their microtubule disruption, whereas platinum-based drugs appear to alter surface ion-channel remodeling initially, and eventually lead to neuronal apoptosis after prolonged exposure [67–69]. Vincristine has also been shown to upregulate the surface expression of 5-hydroxytryptamine2A (5-HT$_{2A}$)receptors in neurons in the dorsal horn and dorsal root ganglion (DRG), sensitizing nociceptors [70]. The development and progression of neuropathies between these three distinct classes of chemotherapeutics are multi-faceted, overlapping in certain aspects, and yet diverse in nature [71].

Painful neuropathies caused by oxaliplatin and paclitaxel share some commonalities of neuronal inflammation, altered ion-channel-expression and excitability of peripheral neurons, and dose-dependent severity [69]. However, while several cellular and molecular markers have been characterized in the development of these distinct neuropathies, the pathophysiology still remains poorly understood [72–74]. Previously, RgIA4 showed antinociceptive efficacy in oxaliplatin-treated rats with dosages as low as 0.128 µg/kg, compared to this study where effects did not become evident until 80 µg/kg [24,25]. In addition, RgIA4 showed a robust reversal of cold allodynia in these oxaliplatin models of CIPN. The reason for these differences is unknown. As such, the differential efficacy of RgIA4 in paclitaxel-treated animals, as compared to previously-reported oxaliplatin-treated animals, may provide a pharmacological tool that can help investigate the distinct, yet intertwining, disease progression between these two pathologies.

Despite the different mechanisms of neuropathology caused by distinct anti-cancer drug classes, the blockade of α9α10 nAChRs appears to be a potential convergent target for the prevention and/or treatment of neuropathic pain across several models. Separate from the α9α10 nAChR subtype, the closely-related homomeric α7 nAChR and the α7β2 nAChR subtypes have been implicated in the modulation of pain. Selective activation of α7 nAChRs with (R)-(-)-3-methoxy-1-oxa-2,7-diaza-7,10-ethanospiro[4.5]dec-2-ene sesquifumarate ((R)-ICH3) or PNU-282987, positive allosteric modulation with GAT107 or PNU-120596, and silent agonism with (R)-N-(4-Methoxyphenyl)-2-((pyridin-3-yloxy)methyl)pi-perazine-1-carboxamide Dihydrochloride (R-47) have shown efficacy in models of inflammatory and neuropathic pain [75–78]. Separately, the α4β2 nAChR agonist (R)-5-(2-azetidinylmethoxy)-2-chloropyridine (ABT-594), an analog inspired by the alkaloid epibatidine isolated from poison arrow frog, *Epipedobates tricolor*, has been shown to result in robust anti-pain effects [79,80]. ABT-594 moved forward into clinical trials but was halted due to adverse side effects.

While chemotherapies are diverse in their mechanisms of action, several drugs across different families have produced similar neuropathies. The use of natural products as a source of therapeutics has proven to be effective but with caveats. Harnessing the evolutionary refinement of these compounds has provided a rich collection of highly specific pharmacological tools. The discovery of paclitaxel was a fortuitous hit from a concerted screening of natural products coordinated by the United States National Cancer Institute looking specifically for compounds that would be efficacious against cancers [3].

Although one of the most widely used chemotherapeutics, the disruptive side effects of paclitaxel are evident. The use of a cone-snail-derived compound as an effective adjuvant treatment highlights the versatility of natural compounds and the importance of continuing the concerted screening and characterization of these molecules for therapeutic applications. The observed efficacy of α9α10 nAChR antagonists in preventing CIPN pain from taxane, platinum-containing, and vinca-alkaloid families of chemotherapeutics suggests a common juncture in the mechanisms of CIPN development across several structural classes of compounds. RgIA4 may be a promising tool in both the treatment of CIPN pain through this mechanism and further characterization of this non-opioid pathway of pain treatment as a molecular probe.

4. Materials and Methods

4.1. Animals

Male Sprague Dawley rats (Envigo) weighing 200–300 g were used in all rat experiments. Rats were housed in groups of two rats per cage with food and water available ad libitum. Animals were maintained in a temperature- and humidity-controlled animal colony maintained on a 12-h light/dark cycle (lights on at 07:00). Male C57BL/6J mice (Jackson Laboratories) were used in all mouse experiments. Mice were housed in groups of four or five per cage with food and water available ad libitum and on the same light cycle. All rat studies were conducted under the approval of the Institutional Animal Care and Use Committee (IACUC) of the University of New England, protocol number 042617-001. All mice experiments were conducted under the approval of the University of Utah IACUC, protocol number 17-08002. The Animal Care and Use Programs and Facilities of the University of Utah are accredited by the Association for Assessment and Accreditation of Laboratory Animal Care (AAALAC) International.

4.2. Drug Solutions and Injections

A clinical formulation of paclitaxel was employed. Paclitaxel USP, extracted from Taxus X media 'Hicksii' (Hospira, IL, USA), came in solution at a concentration of 6 mg/mL. The vehicle used for dilution consisted of 1 part 1:1 Cremophore:EtOH mixture and 2 parts 0.9% saline, and 2 mg/mL sodium citrate. Rats were given a dose of 2 mg/kg (IP) every two days for a total of 4 doses, at a volume of 1 mL/kg body weight. RgIA4 was dissolved in 0.9% saline and injected (SC) once per day, 5 days a week for a total of 15 doses at 1 mL/kg body weight for rats and 4 mL/kg body weight for mice [25]. Upon completion of animal injections, material underwent HPLC analysis to verify its composition and integrity.

4.3. Von Frey Assay

Tactile allodynia was quantified by measuring the hindpaw withdrawal threshold to Von Frey filament stimulation, using the up-down method previously reported [81,82]. Throughout the study, experimenters were blinded to the identity of the injected compound. Rats were divided into treatment groups of $n = 8$ unless otherwise specified. Animals were placed in a clear Plexiglass chamber and allowed to habituate for 15–60 min. Touch-Test filaments (North Coast Medical, Morgan Hill, CA, USA) were used for all testing. For rats, the 2.0 g (4.31) filament was used to start. Clear paw withdrawal, shaking or licking was considered a positive or painful response. This up-down method was stopped four measures after the first positive response. The withdrawal threshold was calculated using the up-down Excel program generously provided by Dr. Michael Ossipov (University of Arizona, Tucson, AZ, USA). The filament range for rats was 3.61, 3.84, 4.08, 4.31, 4.56, 4.74, 4.93, 5.18.

4.4. Plantar Test

Thermal allodynia was quantified by measuring the hindpaw withdrawal latency to noxious radiant heat application in unrestrained animals using the plantar test apparatus (rats: Ugo Basile),

Mar. Drugs **2020**, *18*, 12

as previously reported [83]. Throughout the study, experimenters were blinded to the identity of the injected compound. Rats were divided into treatment groups of $n = 8$ unless otherwise specified. Briefly, animals were placed in a clear Plexiglass chamber and allowed to habituate for 15–60 min. A radiant heat source was then focused on the plantar surface of the hindpaw with the paw withdrawal time automatically determined. The intensity of the heat source was adjusted so that baseline latency was approximately 15 s. A test cutoff time of 30 s was observed to avoid tissue damage.

4.5. Cold Plate

Rats underwent cold plate testing to determine if any sensitivity to cold developed following paclitaxel injection. Throughout the study, experimenters were blinded to the identity of the injected compound. Rats were divided into treatment groups of $n = 8$ unless otherwise specified. A hot/cold plate (Ugo Basile) was used and cooled to 5 °C. To help achieve reliable results a layer of distilled water coated the cold plate. Each rat was placed on the plate, one at a time. The time it took the rat to lick or flick a hind paw or jump to escape the plate was recorded to the nearest 0.1 s. A 5 min cutoff time was used to remove the rat from the plate if they had not yet shown a response to avoid tissue damage.

4.6. Statistical Analysis

In the rat assays, dose- and time-response curves were constructed for each pain model. Mean and standard errors of the mean were calculated. To determine statistical significance either an unpaired *t*-test or two-way ANOVA was performed followed by a Bonferroni posttest using GraphPad Prism software version 6.07 for Windows, GraphPad Software, La Jolla, CA, USA. Significance was established at the $p < 0.05$ level.

Supplementary Materials: The following are available online at http://www.mdpi.com/1660-3397/18/1/12/s1, Figure S1: Paclitaxel did not induce mechanical allodynia in C57BL/6J mice, Figure S2: Tail synaptic nerve action potential (SNAP) conduction velocity was not affected by paclitaxel.

Author Contributions: Conceptualization, methodology, validation, and writing—original draft preparation, review and editing: P.N.H., D.G., K.L.T., S.C., and J.M.M.; formal analysis, investigation, and visualization, P.N.H., D.G., and S.C.; software, P.N.H.; funding acquisition, project administration, and resources, K.L.T. and J.M.M. All authors have read and agreed to the published version of the manuscript.

Funding: This research was supported by the National Institutes of Health (NIH), grant number R01-GM103801 (JMM); the United States Department of Defense, grant number W81XWH1710413 (JMM); and a National Institute of General Medical Sciences (NIGMS) grant, grant number P20GM103643 (D.G., K.L.T.).

Acknowledgments: Special thanks to Doju Yoshikami for helping with the design and assembly of the nerve conduction velocity apparatus and the associated modules made in the LabView software. All rat work was conducted by the University of New England's COBRE Behavior Core and financially supported by NIGMS (grant number P20GM103643).

Conflicts of Interest: The University of Utah holds patents on conopeptides including RgIA4 for which J.M.M. is an inventor. The funders had no role in the design of the study; in the collection, analyses, or interpretation of data; in the writing of the manuscript, or in the decision to publish the results.

Abbreviations

The following abbreviations are used in this manuscript:

ANOVA	Analysis of variance
CCI	Chronic constriction injury
CIPN	Chemotherapy-induced peripheral neuropathy
CNS	Central nervous system
GWAS	Genome-wide association study
IP	Intraperitoneal
nAChR	Nicotinic acetylcholine receptor
NCI	National Cancer Institute
NCV	Nerve conduction velocity
PTX	Paclitaxel

SC	Subcutaneous
SD	Sprague Dawley
SEM	Standard error of the mean
SNAP	Sensory nerve action potential

References

1. van Hecke, O.; Austin, S.K.; Khan, R.A.; Smith, B.H.; Torrance, N. Neuropathic pain in the general population: A systematic review of epidemiological studies. *Pain* **2014**, *155*, 654–662. [CrossRef] [PubMed]
2. Calvo, M.; Dawes, J.M.; Bennett, D.L.H. The role of the immune system in the generation of neuropathic pain. *Lancet Neurol.* **2012**, *11*, 629–642. [CrossRef]
3. Cragg, G.M. Paclitaxel (Taxol®): A success story with valuable lessons for natural product drug discovery and development. *Med. Res. Rev.* **1998**, *18*, 315–331. [CrossRef]
4. Seretny, M.; Currie, G.L.; Sena, E.S.; Ramnarine, S.; Grant, R.; MacLeod, M.R.; Colvin, L.A.; Fallon, M. Incidence, prevalence, and predictors of chemotherapy-induced peripheral neuropathy: A systematic review and meta-analysis. *Pain* **2014**, *155*, 2461–2470. [CrossRef] [PubMed]
5. Song, S.J.; Min, J.; Suh, S.Y.; Jung, S.H.; Hahn, H.J.; Im, S.A.; Lee, J.Y. Incidence of taxane-induced peripheral neuropathy receiving treatment and prescription patterns in patients with breast cancer. *Support. Care Cancer* **2017**, *25*, 2241–2248. [CrossRef] [PubMed]
6. Velasco, R.; Bruna, J. Taxane-Induced Peripheral Neurotoxicity. *Toxics* **2015**, *3*, 152–169. [CrossRef] [PubMed]
7. Dutertre, S.; Jin, A.H.; Vetter, I.; Hamilton, B.; Sunagar, K.; Lavergne, V.; Dutertre, V.; Fry, B.G.; Antunes, A.; Venter, D.J.; et al. Evolution of separate predation- and defence-evoked venoms in carnivorous cone snails. *Nat. Commun.* **2014**, *5*, 3521. [CrossRef] [PubMed]
8. Lewis, R.J.; Dutertre, S.; Vetter, I.; Christie, M.J. Conus venom peptide pharmacology. *Pharm. Rev.* **2012**, *64*, 259–298. [CrossRef] [PubMed]
9. Safavi-Hemami, H.; Gajewiak, J.; Karanth, S.; Robinson, S.D.; Ueberheide, B.; Douglass, A.D.; Schlegel, A.; Imperial, J.S.; Watkins, M.; Bandyopadhyay, P.K.; et al. Specialized insulin is used for chemical warfare by fish-hunting cone snails. *Proc. Natl. Acad. Sci. USA* **2015**, *112*, 1743–1748. [CrossRef] [PubMed]
10. Robinson, S.D.; Li, Q.; Bandyopadhyay, P.K.; Gajewiak, J.; Yandell, M.; Papenfuss, A.T.; Purcell, A.W.; Norton, R.S.; Safavi-Hemami, H. Hormone-like peptides in the venoms of marine cone snails. *Gen. Comp. Endocrinol.* **2017**, *244*, 11–18. [CrossRef]
11. Neves, J.L.; Lin, Z.; Imperial, J.S.; Antunes, A.; Vasconcelos, V.; Olivera, B.M.; Schmidt, E.W. Small Molecules in the Cone Snail Arsenal. *Org. Lett.* **2015**, *17*, 4933–4935. [CrossRef] [PubMed]
12. Dutertre, S.; Jin, A.H.; Kaas, Q.; Jones, A.; Alewood, P.F.; Lewis, R.J. Deep venomics reveals the mechanism for expanded peptide diversity in cone snail venom. *Mol. Cell. Proteom.* **2013**, *12*, 312–329. [CrossRef] [PubMed]
13. Jin, A.H.; Muttenthaler, M.; Dutertre, S.; Himaya, S.W.A.; Kaas, Q.; Craik, D.J.; Lewis, R.J.; Alewood, P.F. Conotoxins: Chemistry and Biology. *Chem. Rev.* **2019**, *119*, 11510–11549. [CrossRef] [PubMed]
14. Pennington, M.W.; Czerwinski, A.; Norton, R.S. Peptide therapeutics from venom: Current status and potential. *Bioorg. Med. Chem.* **2018**, *26*, 2738–2758. [CrossRef] [PubMed]
15. Gao, B.; Peng, C.; Yang, J.; Yi, Y.; Zhang, J.; Shi, Q. Cone Snails: A Big Store of Conotoxins for Novel Drug Discovery. *Toxins* **2017**, *9*, 397. [CrossRef] [PubMed]
16. Giribaldi, J.; Dutertre, S. α-Conotoxins to explore the molecular, physiological and pathophysiological functions of neuronal nicotinic acetylcholine receptors. *Neurosci. Lett.* **2018**, *679*, 24–34. [CrossRef]
17. Green, B.R.; Bulaj, G.; Norton, R.S. Structure and function of mu-conotoxins, peptide-based sodium channel blockers with analgesic activity. *Future Med. Chem.* **2014**, *6*, 1677–1698. [CrossRef]
18. McIntosh, J.M.; Jones, R.M. Cone venom—From accidental stings to deliberate injection. *Toxicon* **2001**, *39*, 1447–1451. [CrossRef]
19. Robinson, S.D.; Norton, R.S. Conotoxin gene superfamilies. *Mar. Drugs* **2014**, *12*, 6058–6101. [CrossRef]
20. Olivera, B.M.; Quik, M.; Vincler, M.; McIntosh, J.M. Subtype-selective conopeptides targeted to nicotinic receptors: Concerted discovery and biomedical applications. *Channels* **2008**, *2*, 143–152. [CrossRef]

21. Ellison, M.; Feng, Z.P.; Park, A.J.; Zhang, X.; Olivera, B.M.; McIntosh, J.M.; Norton, R.S. α-RgIA, a novel conotoxin that blocks the α9α10 nAChR: Structure and identification of key receptor-binding residues. *J. Mol. Biol.* **2008**, *377*, 1216–1227. [CrossRef] [PubMed]

22. Ellison, M.; Haberlandt, C.; Gomez-Casati, M.E.; Watkins, M.; Elgoyhen, A.B.; McIntosh, J.M.; Olivera, B.M. α-RgIA: A novel conotoxin that specifically and potently blocks the α9α10 nAChR. *Biochemistry* **2006**, *45*, 1511–1517. [CrossRef] [PubMed]

23. Azam, L.; Papakyriakou, A.; Zouridakis, M.; Giastas, P.; Tzartos, S.J.; McIntosh, J.M. Molecular interaction of α-conotoxin RgIA with the rat α9α10 nicotinic acetylcholine receptor. *Mol. Pharm.* **2015**, *87*, 855–864. [CrossRef] [PubMed]

24. Christensen, S.B.; Hone, A.J.; Roux, I.; Kniazeff, J.; Pin, J.P.; Upert, G.; Servent, D.; Glowatzki, E.; McIntosh, J.M. RgIA4 Potently Blocks Mouse α9α10 nAChRs and Provides Long Lasting Protection against Oxaliplatin-Induced Cold Allodynia. *Front. Cell. Neurosci.* **2017**, *11*, 219. [CrossRef] [PubMed]

25. Romero, H.K.; Christensen, S.B.; Di Cesare Mannelli, L.; Gajewiak, J.; Ramachandra, R.; Elmslie, K.S.; Vetter, D.E.; Ghelardini, C.; Iadonato, S.P.; Mercado, J.L.; et al. Inhibition of α9α10 nicotinic acetylcholine receptors prevents chemotherapy-induced neuropathic pain. *Proc. Natl. Acad. Sci. USA* **2017**, *114*, E1825–E1832. [CrossRef] [PubMed]

26. Di Cesare Mannelli, L.; Cinci, L.; Micheli, L.; Zanardelli, M.; Pacini, A.; McIntosh, J.M.; Ghelardini, C. α-conotoxin RgIA protects against the development of nerve injury-induced chronic pain and prevents both neuronal and glial derangement. *Pain®* **2014**, *155*, 1986–1995. [CrossRef]

27. Pacini, A.; Micheli, L.; Maresca, M.; Branca, J.J.; McIntosh, J.M.; Ghelardini, C.; Di Cesare Mannelli, L. The α9α10 nicotinic receptor antagonist α-conotoxin RgIA prevents neuropathic pain induced by oxaliplatin treatment. *Exp. Neurol.* **2016**, *282*, 37–48. [CrossRef]

28. Vincler, M.; Wittenauer, S.; Parker, R.; Ellison, M.; Olivera, B.M.; McIntosh, J.M. Molecular mechanism for analgesia involving specific antagonism of α9α10 nicotinic acetylcholine receptors. *Proc. Natl. Acad. Sci. USA* **2006**, *103*, 17880–17884. [CrossRef]

29. Hone, A.J.; McIntosh, J.M. Nicotinic acetylcholine receptors in neuropathic and inflammatory pain. *FEBS Lett.* **2018**, *592*, 1045–1062. [CrossRef]

30. Barrot, M. Tests and models of nociception and pain in rodents. *Neuroscience* **2012**, *211*, 39–50. [CrossRef]

31. Griffiths, L.A.; Duggett, N.A.; Pitcher, A.L.; Flatters, S.J.L. Evoked and Ongoing Pain-Like Behaviours in a Rat Model of Paclitaxel-Induced Peripheral Neuropathy. *Pain Res. Manag.* **2018**, *2018*, 8217613. [CrossRef] [PubMed]

32. Smith, S.B.; Crager, S.E.; Mogil, J.S. Paclitaxel-induced neuropathic hypersensitivity in mice: Responses in 10 inbred mouse strains. *Life Sci.* **2004**, *74*, 2593–2604. [CrossRef] [PubMed]

33. Makker, P.G.; Duffy, S.S.; Lees, J.G.; Perera, C.J.; Tonkin, R.S.; Butovsky, O.; Park, S.B.; Goldstein, D.; Moalem-Taylor, G. Characterisation of Immune and Neuroinflammatory Changes Associated with Chemotherapy-Induced Peripheral Neuropathy. *PLoS ONE* **2017**, *12*, e0170814. [CrossRef] [PubMed]

34. Marmiroli, P.; Riva, B.; Pozzi, E.; Ballarini, E.; Lim, D.; Chiorazzi, A.; Meregalli, C.; Distasi, C.; Renn, C.L.; Semperboni, S.; et al. Susceptibility of different mouse strains to oxaliplatin peripheral neurotoxicity: Phenotypic and genotypic insights. *PLoS ONE* **2017**, *12*, e0186250. [CrossRef] [PubMed]

35. Chua, K.C.; Kroetz, D.L. Genetic advances uncover mechanisms of chemotherapy-induced peripheral neuropathy. *Clin Pharm. Ther.* **2017**, *101*, 450–452. [CrossRef] [PubMed]

36. Park, S.B.; Lin, C.S.; Krishnan, A.V.; Goldstein, D.; Friedlander, M.L.; Kiernan, M.C. Oxaliplatin-induced neurotoxicity: Changes in axonal excitability precede development of neuropathy. *Brain* **2009**, *132*, 2712–2723. [CrossRef] [PubMed]

37. Sittl, R.; Lampert, A.; Huth, T.; Schuy, E.T.; Link, A.S.; Fleckenstein, J.; Alzheimer, C.; Grafe, P.; Carr, R.W. Anticancer drug oxaliplatin induces acute cooling-aggravated neuropathy via sodium channel subtype Na(V)1.6-resurgent and persistent current. *Proc. Natl. Acad. Sci. USA* **2012**, *109*, 6704–6709. [CrossRef]

38. Augusto, C.; Pietro, M.; Cinzia, M.; Sergio, C.; Sara, C.; Luca, G.; Scaioli, V. Peripheral neuropathy due to paclitaxel: Study of the temporal relationships between the therapeutic schedule and the clinical quantitative score (QST) and comparison with neurophysiological findings. *J. Neurooncol.* **2008**, *86*, 89–99. [CrossRef]

39. Alushin, G.M.; Lander, G.C.; Kellogg, E.H.; Zhang, R.; Baker, D.; Nogales, E. High-resolution microtubule structures reveal the structural transitions in αβ-tubulin upon GTP hydrolysis. *Cell* **2014**, *157*, 1117–1129. [CrossRef]

40. Bandos, H.; Melnikow, J.; Rivera, D.R.; Swain, S.M.; Sturtz, K.; Fehrenbacher, L.; Wade, J.L., III; Brufsky, A.M.; Julian, T.B.; Margolese, R.G.; et al. Long-term Peripheral Neuropathy in Breast Cancer Patients Treated With Adjuvant Chemotherapy: NRG Oncology/NSABP B-30. *J. Natl. Cancer Inst.* **2018**, *110*, djx162. [CrossRef]

41. Rivera, D.R.; Ganz, P.A.; Weyrich, M.S.; Bandos, H.; Melnikow, J. Chemotherapy-Associated Peripheral Neuropathy in Patients With Early-Stage Breast Cancer: A Systematic Review. *J. Natl. Cancer Inst.* **2018**, *110*, djx140. [CrossRef] [PubMed]

42. van den Bent, M.J.; van Raaij-van den Aarssen, V.J.; Verweij, J.; Doorn, P.A.; Sillevis Smitt, P.A. Progression of paclitaxel-induced neuropathy following discontinuation of treatment. *Muscle Nerve* **1997**, *20*, 750–752. [CrossRef]

43. Satkunanathan, N.; Livett, B.; Gayler, K.; Sandall, D.; Down, J.; Khalil, Z. Alpha-conotoxin Vc1.1 alleviates neuropathic pain and accelerates functional recovery of injured neurones. *Brain Res.* **2005**, *1059*, 149–158. [CrossRef] [PubMed]

44. Andrade, A.; Denome, S.; Jiang, Y.Q.; Marangoudakis, S.; Lipscombe, D. Opioid inhibition of N-type Ca2+ channels and spinal analgesia couple to alternative splicing. *Nat. Neurosci.* **2010**, *13*, 1249–1256. [CrossRef] [PubMed]

45. Seward, E.; Hammond, C.; Henderson, G. Mu-opioid-receptor-mediated inhibition of the N-type calcium-channel current. *Proc. Biol. Sci.* **1991**, *244*, 129–135. [PubMed]

46. Tedford, H.W.; Zamponi, G.W. Direct G protein modulation of Cav2 calcium channels. *Pharm. Rev.* **2006**, *58*, 837–862. [CrossRef]

47. Berecki, G.; McArthur, J.R.; Cuny, H.; Clark, R.J.; Adams, D.J. Differential Cav2.1 and Cav2.3 channel inhibition by baclofen and α-conotoxin Vc1.1 via GABAB receptor activation. *J. Gen. Physiol.* **2014**, *143*, 465–479. [CrossRef]

48. Callaghan, B.; Haythornthwaite, A.; Berecki, G.; Clark, R.J.; Craik, D.J.; Adams, D.J. Analgesic α-conotoxins Vc1.1 and Rg1A inhibit N-type calcium channels in rat sensory neurons via GABAB receptor activation. *J. Neurosci.* **2008**, *28*, 10943–10951. [CrossRef]

49. Castro, J.; Harrington, A.M.; Garcia-Caraballo, S.; Maddern, J.; Grundy, L.; Zhang, J.; Page, G.; Miller, P.E.; Craik, D.J.; Adams, D.J.; et al. α-Conotoxin Vc1.1 inhibits human dorsal root ganglion neuroexcitability and mouse colonic nociception via GABAB receptors. *Gut* **2017**, *66*, 1083–1094. [CrossRef]

50. Huynh, T.G.; Cuny, H.; Slesinger, P.A.; Adams, D.J. Novel mechanism of voltage-gated N-type (Cav2.2) calcium channel inhibition revealed through α-conotoxin Vc1.1 activation of the GABA(B) receptor. *Mol. Pharm.* **2015**, *87*, 240–250. [CrossRef]

51. Mohammadi, S.; Christie, M.J. α9-nicotinic acetylcholine receptors contribute to the maintenance of chronic mechanical hyperalgesia, but not thermal or mechanical allodynia. *Mol. Pain* **2014**, *10*, 64. [CrossRef] [PubMed]

52. Mohammadi, S.A.; Christie, M.J. Conotoxin Interactions with α9α10-nAChRs: Is the α9α10-Nicotinic Acetylcholine Receptor an Important Therapeutic Target for Pain Management? *Toxins* **2015**, *7*, 3916–3932. [CrossRef] [PubMed]

53. Peng, H.; Ferris, R.L.; Matthews, T.; Hiel, H.; Lopez-Albaitero, A.; Lustig, L.R. Characterization of the human nicotinic acetylcholine receptor subunit alpha (α) 9 (CHRNA9) and alpha (α) 10 (CHRNA10) in lymphocytes. *Life Sci.* **2004**, *76*, 263–280. [CrossRef] [PubMed]

54. Richter, K.; Mathes, V.; Fronius, M.; Althaus, M.; Hecker, A.; Krasteva-Christ, G.; Padberg, W.; Hone, A.J.; McIntosh, J.M.; Zakrzewicz, A.; et al. Phosphocholine—An agonist of metabotropic but not of ionotropic functions of α9-containing nicotinic acetylcholine receptors. *Sci. Rep.* **2016**, *6*, 28660. [CrossRef] [PubMed]

55. Zheng, G.; Zhang, Z.; Dowell, C.; Wala, E.; Dwoskin, L.P.; Holtman, J.R.; McIntosh, J.M.; Crooks, P.A. Discovery of non-peptide, small molecule antagonists of α9α10 nicotinic acetylcholine receptors as novel analgesics for the treatment of neuropathic and tonic inflammatory pain. *Bioorg. Med. Chem. Lett.* **2011**, *21*, 2476–2479. [CrossRef] [PubMed]

56. Wala, E.P.; Crooks, P.A.; McIntosh, J.M.; Holtman, J.R., Jr. Novel small molecule α9α10 nicotinic receptor antagonist prevents and reverses chemotherapy-evoked neuropathic pain in rats. *Anesth. Analg.* **2012**, *115*, 713–720. [CrossRef] [PubMed]

57. Holtman, J.R.; Dwoskin, L.P.; Dowell, C.; Wala, E.P.; Zhang, Z.; Crooks, P.A.; McIntosh, J.M. The novel small molecule α9α10 nicotinic acetylcholine receptor antagonist ZZ-204G is analgesic. *Eur. J. Pharm.* **2011**, *670*, 500–508. [CrossRef]

58. Li, X.; Hu, Y.; Wu, Y.; Huang, Y.; Yu, S.; Ding, Q.; Zhangsun, D.; Luo, S. Anti-hypersensitive effect of intramuscular administration of αO-conotoxin GeXIVA[1,2] and GeXIVA[1,4] in rats of neuropathic pain. *Prog. Neuropsychopharmacol. Biol. Psychiatry* **2016**, *66*, 112–119. [CrossRef]

59. Luo, S.; Zhangsun, D.; Harvey, P.J.; Kaas, Q.; Wu, Y.; Zhu, X.; Hu, Y.; Li, X.; Tsetlin, V.I.; Christensen, S.; et al. Cloning, synthesis, and characterization of αO-conotoxin GeXIVA, a potent α9α10 nicotinic acetylcholine receptor antagonist. *Proc. Natl. Acad. Sci. USA* **2015**, *112*, E4026–E4035. [CrossRef]

60. Wang, H.; Li, X.; Zhangsun, D.; Yu, G.; Su, R.; Luo, S. The α9α10 Nicotinic Acetylcholine Receptor Antagonist αO-Conotoxin GeXIVA[1,2] Alleviates and Reverses Chemotherapy-Induced Neuropathic Pain. *Mar. Drugs* **2019**, *17*, 265. [CrossRef]

61. Santos, A.D.; McIntosh, J.M.; Hillyard, D.R.; Cruz, L.J.; Olivera, B.M. The A-superfamily of conotoxins: Structural and functional divergence. *J. Biol. Chem.* **2004**, *279*, 17596–17606. [CrossRef] [PubMed]

62. Jordan, M.A.; Wilson, L. Microtubules as a target for anticancer drugs. *Nat. Rev. Cancer* **2004**, *4*, 253–265. [CrossRef] [PubMed]

63. Pazdur, R.; Kudelka, A.P.; Kavanagh, J.J.; Cohen, P.R.; Raber, M.N. The taxoids: Paclitaxel (Taxol) and docetaxel (Taxotere). *Cancer Treat. Rev.* **1993**, *19*, 351–386. [CrossRef]

64. Tangutur, A.D.; Kumar, D.; Krishna, K.V.; Kantevari, S. Microtubule Targeting Agents as Cancer Chemotherapeutics: An Overview of Molecular Hybrids as Stabilizing and Destabilizing Agents. *Curr. Top Med. Chem.* **2017**, *17*, 2523–2537. [CrossRef] [PubMed]

65. Jordan, M. Mechanism of Action of Antitumor Drugs that Interact with Microtubules and Tubulin. *Curr. Med. Chem. Anti-Cancer Agents* **2012**, *2*, 1–17. [CrossRef]

66. Raymond, E.; Faivre, S.; Chaney, S.; Woynarowski, J.; Cvitkovic, E. Cellular and Molecular Pharmacology of Oxalipaltin. *Mol. Cancer Ther.* **2002**, *1*, 227–235.

67. Brewer, J.R.; Morrison, G.; Dolan, M.E.; Fleming, G.F. Chemotherapy-induced peripheral neuropathy: Current status and progress. *Gynecol. Oncol.* **2016**, *140*, 176–183. [CrossRef]

68. Descoeur, J.; Pereira, V.; Pizzoccaro, A.; Francois, A.; Ling, B.; Maffre, V.; Couette, B.; Busserolles, J.; Courteix, C.; Noel, J.; et al. Oxaliplatin-induced cold hypersensitivity is due to remodelling of ion channel expression in nociceptors. *EMBO Mol. Med.* **2011**, *3*, 266–278. [CrossRef]

69. Zajaczkowska, R.; Kocot-Kepska, M.; Leppert, W.; Wrzosek, A.; Mika, J.; Wordliczek, J. Mechanisms of Chemotherapy-Induced Peripheral Neuropathy. *Int. J. Mol. Sci.* **2019**, *20*, 1451. [CrossRef]

70. Thibault, K.; Van Steenwinckel, J.; Brisorgueil, M.J.; Fischer, J.; Hamon, M.; Calvino, B.; Conrath, M. Serotonin 5-HT2A receptor involvement and Fos expression at the spinal level in vincristine-induced neuropathy in the rat. *Pain* **2008**, *140*, 305–322. [CrossRef]

71. Jaggi, A.S.; Singh, N. Mechanisms in cancer-chemotherapeutic drugs-induced peripheral neuropathy. *Toxicol.* **2012**, *291*, 1–9. [CrossRef] [PubMed]

72. Flatters, S.J.L.; Dougherty, P.M.; Colvin, L.A. Clinical and preclinical perspectives on Chemotherapy-Induced Peripheral Neuropathy (CIPN): A narrative review. *Br. J. Anaesth.* **2017**, *119*, 737–749. [CrossRef] [PubMed]

73. Starobova, H.; Vetter, I. Pathophysiology of Chemotherapy-Induced Peripheral Neuropathy. *Front. Mol. Neurosci.* **2017**, *10*, 174. [CrossRef] [PubMed]

74. Dougherty, P.M.; Cata, J.P.; Cordella, J.V.; Burton, A.; Weng, H.R. Taxol-induced sensory disturbance is characterized by preferential impairment of myelinated fiber function in cancer patients. *Pain* **2004**, *109*, 132–142. [CrossRef] [PubMed]

75. Bagdas, D.; Wilkerson, J.L.; Kulkarni, A.; Toma, W.; AlSharari, S.; Gul, Z.; Lichtman, A.H.; Papke, R.L.; Thakur, G.A.; Damaj, M.I. The α7 nicotinic receptor dual allosteric agonist and positive allosteric modulator GAT107 reverses nociception in mouse models of inflammatory and neuropathic pain. *Br. J. Pharm.* **2016**, *173*, 2506–2520. [CrossRef]

76. Damaj, M.I.; Meyer, E.M.; Martin, B.R. The antinociceptive effects of α7 nicotinic agonists in an acute pain model. *Neuropharmacology* **2000**, *39*, 2785–2791. [CrossRef]

77. Freitas, K.; Ghosh, S.; Ivy Carroll, F.; Lichtman, A.H.; Imad Damaj, M. Effects of α7 positive allosteric modulators in murine inflammatory and chronic neuropathic pain models. *Neuropharmacology* **2013**, *65*, 156–164. [CrossRef]

78. Toma, W.; Kyte, S.L.; Bagdas, D.; Jackson, A.; Meade, J.A.; Rahman, F.; Chen, Z.J.; Del Fabbro, E.; Cantwell, L.; Kulkarni, A.; et al. The α7 nicotinic receptor silent agonist R-47 prevents and reverses paclitaxel-induced peripheral neuropathy in mice without tolerance or altering nicotine reward and withdrawal. *Exp. Neurol.* **2019**, *320*, 113010. [CrossRef]

79. Di Cesare Mannelli, L.; Pacini, A.; Matera, C.; Zanardelli, M.; Mello, T.; De Amici, M.; Dallanoce, C.; Ghelardini, C. Involvement of α7 nAChR subtype in rat oxaliplatin-induced neuropathy: Effects of selective activation. *Neuropharmacology* **2014**, *79*, 37–48. [CrossRef]

80. Rowbotham, M.C.; Duan, W.R.; Thomas, J.; Nothaft, W.; Backonja, M.M. A randomized, double-blind, placebo-controlled trial evaluating the efficacy and safety of ABT-594 in patients with diabetic peripheral neuropathic pain. *Pain* **2009**, *146*, 245–252. [CrossRef]

81. Chaplan, S.R.; Bach, F.W.; Pogrel, J.W.; Chung, J.M.; Yaksh, T.L. Quantitative assessment of tactile allodynia in the rat paw. *J. Neurosci. Methods* **1994**, *53*, 55–63. [CrossRef]

82. Dixon, W.J. Efficient analysis of experimental observations. *Annu. Rev. Pharm. Toxicol.* **1980**, *20*, 441–462. [CrossRef] [PubMed]

83. Hargreaves, K.; Dubner, R.; Brown, F.; Flores, C.; Joris, J. A new and sensitive method for measuring thermal nociception in cutaneous hyperalgesia. *Pain* **1988**, *32*, 77–88. [CrossRef]

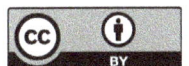

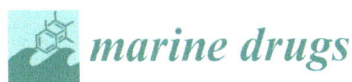

Article

Venomics Reveals Venom Complexity of the Piscivorous Cone Snail, *Conus tulipa*

Mriga Dutt [1], Sébastien Dutertre [2], Ai-Hua Jin [1], Vincent Lavergne [3], Paul Francis Alewood [1] and Richard James Lewis [1,*]

[1] Institute for Molecular Bioscience, The University of Queensland, St. Lucia, Queensland 4068, Australia; m.dutt@uq.edu.au (M.D.); a.jin@imb.uq.edu.au (A.-H.J.); p.alewood@imb.uq.edu.au (P.F.A.)
[2] Institut des Biomolecules Max Mousseron, UMR 5247, Université Montpellier-CNRS, 34093 Montpellier, France; sebastien.dutertre@umontpellier.fr
[3] Léon Bérard Cancer Center, 28 rue Laennec, 69008 Lyon, France; vincent.lavergne@lyon.unicancer.fr
* Correspondence: r.lewis@imb.uq.edu.au; Tel.: +61-07-3346-2984

Received: 4 December 2018; Accepted: 14 January 2019; Published: 21 January 2019

Abstract: The piscivorous cone snail *Conus tulipa* has evolved a net-hunting strategy, akin to the deadly *Conus geographus*, and is considered the second most dangerous cone snail to humans. Here, we present the first venomics study of *C. tulipa* venom using integrated transcriptomic and proteomic approaches. Parallel transcriptomic analysis of two *C. tulipa* specimens revealed striking differences in conopeptide expression levels (2.5-fold) between individuals, identifying 522 and 328 conotoxin precursors from 18 known gene superfamilies. Despite broad overlap at the superfamily level, only 86 precursors (11%) were common to both specimens. Conantokins (NMDA antagonists) from the superfamily B1 dominated the transcriptome and proteome of *C. tulipa* venom, along with superfamilies B2, A, O1, O3, con-ikot-ikot and conopressins, plus novel putative conotoxins precursors T1.3, T6.2, T6.3, T6.4 and T8.1. Thus, *C. tulipa* venom comprised both paralytic (putative ion channel modulating α-, ω-, μ-, δ-) and non-paralytic (conantokins, con-ikot-ikots, conopressins) conotoxins. This venomic study confirms the potential for non-paralytic conotoxins to contribute to the net-hunting strategy of *C. tulipa*.

Keywords: conotoxin; *Conus tulipa*; intraspecific variation; venomics; transcriptomics; proteomics; conantokins; net hunting strategy; nirvana cabal; ion channel modulators

1. Introduction

Venomous animals have long been regarded as a valuable source of bioactive peptides that can have therapeutic potential, with several currently used clinically [1–4]. Marine cone snails produce relatively short cysteine-rich bioactive peptides called conotoxins that target various ion channels and receptors [5]. Amongst animal venoms, conotoxins arguably display the broadest suite of posttranslational modifications (PTM), which contribute to the broad spectrum of bioactivity in these exceptionally potent venoms [6]. To date, more than 800 species of snails in the genus *Conus* have been documented [7] with most species producing in excess of 1000 conotoxins [8]. As these molluscs are sluggish and small, it is clear that their complex venom arsenal has contributed to their success as predators [9,10]. To accelerate conotoxin discovery, there has been a shift from traditional assay-guided fractionation and Sanger sequencing to an increased use of next-generation sequencing (NGS) and proteomics as part of an integrated "venomics" approach [11]. Venomics has contributed to recent breakthrough in our understanding of the ecology and evolution of cone snails, including the role of defence in diet diversification [12] and biological messiness [13–16] in the accelerated diversification of conopeptides.

Cone snail venom composition appears to be affected by geography, diet and season [17], however, significant differences between individuals of the same species [8,18–21] make comparisons difficult and many earlier studies using pooled venom samples ignored the importance of venom variability [22]. Most well-studied *Conus* venoms have been isolated from fish hunting species that have evolved to target vertebrates [5,23]. The piscivorous cone snail *Conus tulipa* is classified phylogenetically in the *Gastridium* clade along with the closely related and potentially lethal *Conus geographus* [24]. Whereas this study follows the phylogeny published by Puillandre et al. [7], where the *Gastridium* species represents a subgenus within the single genus *Conus*, other authors have suggested that *Gastridium* should be recognized as a separate genus [25]. *C. tulipa* (50–80 mm) is smaller than *C. geographus* (80–120mm) but both possess a thin fragile shell and are generally considered the deadliest cone snails to humans [24]. Nevertheless, no systematic characterization of *C. tulipa* venom has been reported, with only ρ-TIA [26–28], μ-TIIIA [29], conantokin-T [30], conotoxin TVIIA [31] and conopressin-T [32] characterized to date. *C. tulipa* utilises a net-feeding strategy, exclusive to this clade, which involves enlargement of the snail's rostrum and secretion of conotoxin(s) presumably through the proboscis to suppress the escape response of fish facilitating prey capture by mouth. Olivera et al. coined the 'nirvana cabal' [22] to describe the chemistry that facilitates net feeding, although the bioactive components of the nirvana cabal remain to be fully characterized.

Using 454 pyrosequencing combined with top-down and bottom-up mass spectrometry and dedicated bioinformatic tools, we characterized the complex mixture of venom peptides that comprise the venom of *C. tulipa*. Insights into intraspecific venom peptides were obtained by comparing the transcriptomes of two specimens of *C. tulipa* collected from the same geographical location. This systematic characterization broadens our understanding of the venom peptides contributing to the predatory and defensive behaviour of *C. tulipa*.

2. Results

2.1. Transcriptomic Intraspecific Variation

Using 454 sequencing, ConoSorter and manual editing, we generated venom gland transcriptome databases for two *C. tulipa* specimens, S1 and S2. The S1 intact venom duct yielded 522 conotoxin precursors that clustered into 16 known gene superfamilies (Table S1), while stripped venom duct of S2 yielded fewer (328) conotoxin precursors that clustered into 18 known gene superfamilies (Table 1 and Table S1). Overall, 16 gene superfamilies were common to both specimens (Table 1, Figure 1), with superfamily B1 encoding conantokins dominating the venom gland transcriptome of both specimens. In addition, gene superfamilies B2, O1, O3, con-ikot-ikot, conopressins and conoporins had high expression levels in both specimens (Figure 1). No novel gene superfamily was identified.

Table 1. Transcriptomic variation between two *C. tulipa* specimens.

Transcriptome Features	Specimen 1 (S1)	Specimen 2 (S2)
454 raw reads generated	100,564	33,516
Number of final conotoxin precursors	522	328
Number of gene superfamilies	16	18
Total read frequency (level of transcription)	16,333	6426

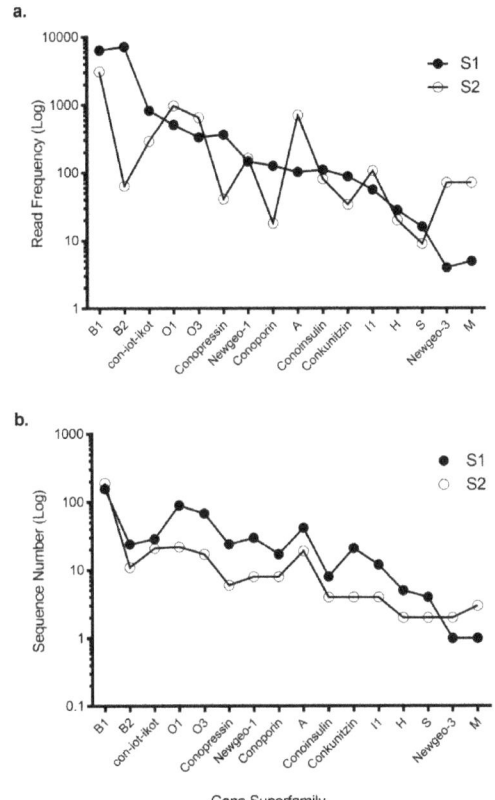

Figure 1. Transcriptomic expression of gene superfamilies for S1 and S2. (**a**) The conopeptide precursor read frequency and (**b**) the number of unique conotoxin sequences expressed by each specimen across the 16 common gene superfamilies. These data highlight the variable read frequency, with S1 expressing significantly more unique sequences across all superfamilies except the newgeo-3 and M superfamilies.

Eighty-six conotoxin precursors (Tu001–Tu086) were common to both specimens, comprising ~ 10% of the total identified conotoxin precursors. Of these, 29 belonged to B1, 2 to B2, 11 to O1, 6 to O3, 8 to A, 8 to con-ikot-ikot, 4 to conopressin-conophysin and 6 to the recently described newgeo-1 superfamily from *C. geographus* (Table S2). Interestingly, most precursors had widely varying read frequencies between the specimens. For example, precursor Tu029 was the highest expressing superfamily B1 precursor in S1 (162 reads) but one of the lowest expressing (2 reads) in S2. In contrast, precursor Tu020 was highly expressed in S2 (495 reads) but had only 12 reads in S1 (Figure 2). Overall, 41 of 86 common conotoxin precursors had read levels that were within 3-fold difference (Table S2).

a.

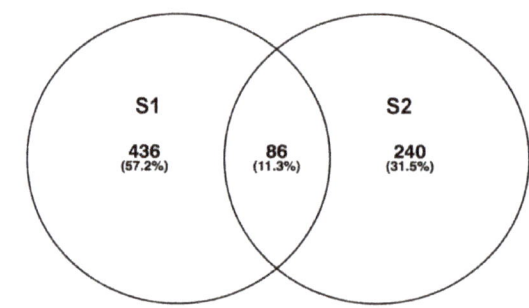

b.

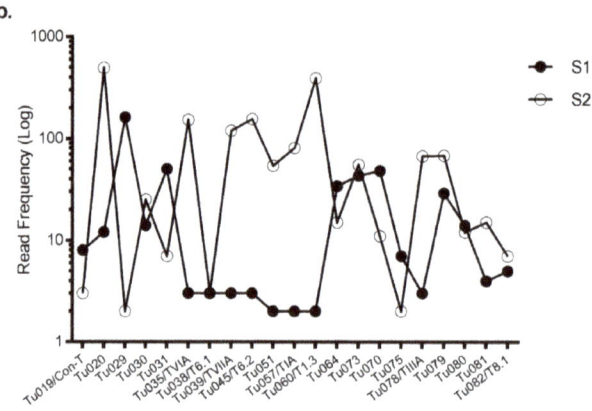

Figure 2. Expression of common precursors in S1 and S2. **(a)** A Venn diagram representing the total number of precursors found in S1 and S2. Both specimens commonly expressed 86 conopeptide precursors. **(b)** Expression level of the common precursors in S1 and S2. For superfamilies that shared >10 precursors (eg, B1, O1, O3), data is shown for the highest expressing precursor for each specimen in that superfamily. For known venom peptides, their name follows the transcript nomenclature.

2.2. Proteome Analysis

LC-MS analysis was performed on the proximal (P), proximal central (PC), distal central (DC) and distal (D) sections of the S2 venom duct (Figure 3). The P and PC sections had similar profiles, with twelve common masses shared between the two sections. In contrast, the DC and D sections were each quite distinct, with the DC section producing only a few easily detectable masses, while the D section was more complex. Through a combined top-down and bottom-up proteomics approaches, we confirmed the presence of 7 of 9 reported *C. tulipa* venom peptides (Table S3). These include ρ-TIA (2389.22 Da), conopressin-T (1107.567 Da) and T1.1 (1904.249 Da) in the P and PC sections (Figure 3), though low levels of the former were also identified in the DC section (Figure 4). In the D section, the dominant mass was conantokin-T (2682.351 Da) and the moderately expressing T1.2 (1953.246 Da) (Figure 4). Tandem MS/MS analysis of the duct sections detected and confirmed the presence of 18 conotoxins (Table 2).

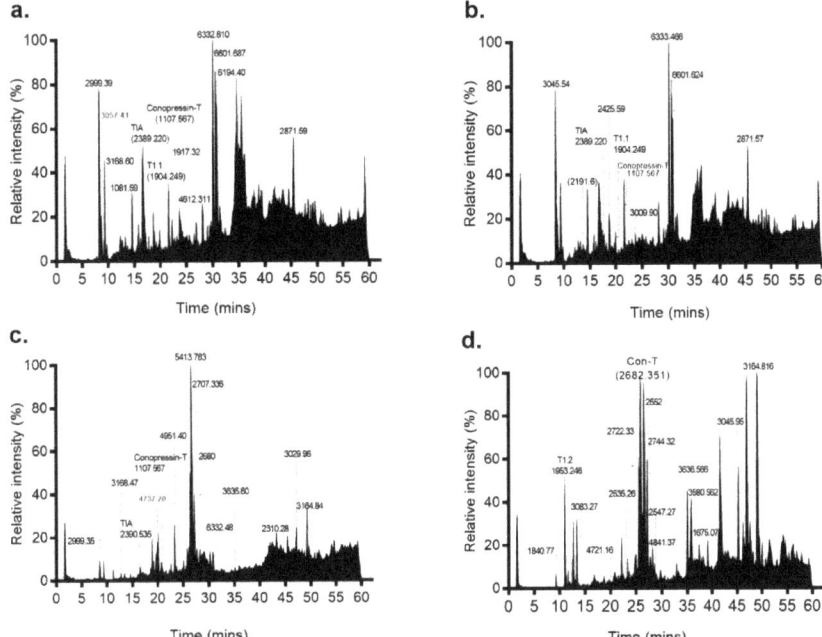

Figure 3. Mass profiles of the four venom duct segments of *C. tulipa*. LC-MS profiles of (**a**) proximal, (**b**) proximal central, (**c**) distal central and (**d**) distal sections of the venom duct are shown, with prominent masses indicated. The mass profiles for the proximal and proximal central sections were similar and included three known conotoxins ρ-TIA (relative intensity 10.2%), T1.1 (relative intensity 0.17%) and conopressin-T (relative intensity 57.5%). In contrast, the mass profiles for the distal and distal central sections are quite different, with the latter displaying a much simpler peptide profile dominated by the peptide mass 5413.783 Da, while the distal section was dominated by Con-T (2682.351 Da) along with peptide masses 2722.33 Da, 2744.32 Da and T1.2. Additionally, relatively low expression of conopressin-T (4.45%) and ρ-TIA (0.1%) peptides was observed within the DC section.

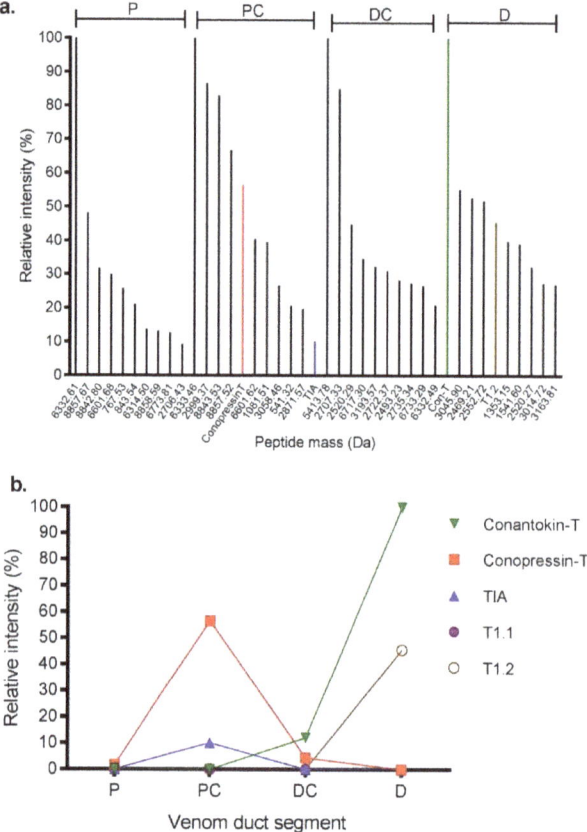

Figure 4. Relative intensity of prominent venom peptides expressed in different sections of the *C. tulipa* venom duct. **(a)** Relative intensity of the ten dominant peptides from the proximal (P), proximal central (PC), distal central (DC), and distal (D) venom duct sections. Conopressin-T (red bar), ρ-TIA (blue bar) and conantokin-T (green bar) were amongst the major expressing peptides analysed in the proteome **(b)** Relative intensity of known *C. tulipa* peptide masses across the venom duct sections. Conantokin-T (2682. 3514 Da) dominated the D section, while conopressin-T (1107. 5675 Da) and ρ-TIA (2389.2206 Da) had relatively high expression levels in the PC sections. T1.2 (1953.2469 Da) also had relatively high expression in the D section, while T1.1 (1904.2497 Da) showed relatively low expression across the venom duct.

Table 2. Novel conotoxin precursors identified in the four venom duct sections of *C. tulipa* by LC-MS/MS at 99% confidence.

[1] Section	Matched Precursor (S2)	MS/MS Fragment	PTM	Precursor (Da)	z
D	Tu0051/T1.2	SNPA⊂AGNNPH	Ala->Gly@5	1169.430	2
D	Tu316	AIASSVVTPGSSMK		1333.691	2
D	Tu068	MINAETQTR		1062.510	2
D	Tu065	NCMLINVQQLGLR	Asn -> Thr @1, carbamidometh@2	1544.830	2
D	Tu020	MLENLREAEVK	Carboxy(E)@3	1374.681	3
D	Tu076	ADRDTDPDDENPR	Oxidation(P)@7	1530.618	3
DC	Tu056/T1.3	VKDFK		635.364	2
DC	Tu316	AIASSVVTPGSSMK		1333.691	2
DC	Tu065	NCMLINVQQLGLR		1524.820	2
DC	Tu068	MINAETQTR		1062.500	2
DC	Tu314	DLADTRYR	Arg -> Ser @ 6	939.4289	2
DC	Tu320	AAFHMFYFDQFSK		1637.730	3
PC	Tu298/T6.4	DGTGQCAPK	Gln->Asp@5, Carbamydomethyl @ 8, oxid(P)@10,	1190.560	3
PC	Tu297/T6.4	VFDNR		658.351	2
PC	Tu032/T6.1	DALKNLK		800.457	2
PC	Tu035/TVIA	SCNPYSR	Carbamydomethi@2, Deamidated(N)@3, Oxidation(P)@4,	899.342	2
PC	Tu274/TVIA	ALKNLKDSRGGSAR	Deamidated(R)@8.	1474.787	2
PC	Tu314	VVTSGSSLQGTSLK		1362.730	2
PC	Tu075	VFIYGGCDGNANR		1428.640	2
PC	Tu316	AIASSVVTPGSSMK		1333.690	2
PC	Tu059/conopressin-T	NLDMIEGH		910.413	2
PC	Tu296/T6.4	VRDNR		658.340	2
PC	Tu314	GIASKVVTSGSSLQ		1332.830	2
PC	Tu030	VPEDASMLQGFDQG		1475.780	2
P	Tu030	LPFNNVEGATNDLGJFEPSAENEDGKFRFF	Deam @ 3	1475.650	2
P	Tu076	LTL5APK		728.443	2
P	Tu075	AAFHMFYFDQFSK		1637.735	3
P	Tu059/conopressin-T	NLDMIEGH		910.414	2
P	Tu314	FALKNPVLQINSCVTTSTPTGIEPGK	Deamidated(N)@5; Deamidated(N)@11; Ser->Gly@12	2640.405	3
P	Tu314	AVRAIASSVVTPGSSMKGGPLK		2112.360	3
P	Tu314	VVTSGSSLQGTSLKDLADTRYRVTCAIQVENWTK		2321.149	3

[1] Distal (D), Distal Central (DC), Proximal Central (PC) and Proximal (P).

2.3. Transcriptomic Variance Within Gene Superfamilies

2.3.1. Superfamily B1 [33]

Superfamily B1 dominated expression in both the specimens, with a total of 377 precursors recovered, including 157 unique precursors in S1 and 191 unique precursors in S2, together with 29 common precursors (Tu001–Tu029). Conantokin-T has been well-characterized [33] but its gene precursor sequence has remained incomplete. From our transcriptome analysis, we established the full precursor sequence of conantokin-T (Tu020), with most other B1 superfamily transcripts being variants of conantokin-T (Table S1). MS/MS analysis matched peptide fragments belonging to Tu020 (495 reads) from S2 found in the distal venom duct, confirming venom expression of conantokin-T (2682.35 Da) (Table 2).

2.3.2. Superfamily B2 [14]

In *C. tulipa*, twenty-four B2 precursors were identified in the transcriptome of S1 at moderate transcription levels. Of the thirteen precursors identified in S2, MS/MS analysis only detected fragments belonging to a single conotoxin precursor (Tu030, 25 reads) found in the PC and P sections of the venom duct (Table 2). B2 peptides are cysteine poor, similar to the superfamily B1 conantokins (Table S4). Only two B2 conotoxin precursors (Tu030 and Tu031) were common to both specimens (Table S2).

2.3.3. Superfamily O1 [34]

S1 and S2 expressed 83 and 11 unique superfamily O1 precursors, respectively, with eleven precursors (Tu032–Tu042) common to both specimens (Table S2). The O1 precursors expressed in S1 and S2 could be classified into four major subtypes based on their propeptide sequences, including precursors for TVIA, TVIIA, putative T6.1 and a putative new peptide sequence named T6.2 (Table S4). Despite 23 precursors encoding for TVIA in S1 and 7 in S2, only two precursors (Tu034 and Tu035) were common to both (Table S2). For TVIIA, we found two precursors common to both S1 and S2. The MS/MS analysis detected fragments matching to two precursors encoding for TVIA (Tu035, 153 reads and Tu274, 376 reads) and a fragment matching precursor encoding for a putative T6.1 toxin (Tu032, 3 reads) in the PC section (Table 2).

2.3.4. Superfamily O3 [35]

Fifty-eight unique superfamily O3 precursors from S1 and 12 from S2 were identified, while six precursors (Tu043–Tu048) were common to both specimens. All precursors had the same signal sequence MSGLGIMVLTLLLLVLMTTSH, and depending on their mature peptide sequence differences, superfamily O3 precursors were classified into two groups; T6.3 (SAKGTVSWRKKHCCCIRSNGPKCSRICIFKFWC) that displayed 92% similarity to G20 [35], and T6.4 (CEMQCEQKKKHCCRVREERIQCAPKCWGIEW) that was 90% similar to G6.6 (Table S4) [32]. MS/MS fragments matching two T6.4 precursors (Tu297, 51 reads and Tu298, 76 reads) were detected in the PC venom duct sections of S2 (Table 2).

2.3.5. Superfamily A [36]

S1 expressed thirty-three unique superfamily A precursors and S2 eleven unique precursors, with eight precursors (Tu049-Tu056) common to both (Table S2). Superfamily A conopeptides included ρ-conotoxin TIA and putative α-conotoxins T1.1 and T1.2 (Table S4). Broadly, the analysed precursors could be classified into four subgroups depending on their mature sequence, (Table S4). The new peptide T1.3 (Tu056, 391 reads) displayed high similarity to peptide G1.9 from *C. geographus* [37], with MS/MS detecting a fragment matching T1.3 in the DC venom duct section (Table 2). 15 ρ-TIA precursors from S1 and two from S2 were detected, with S1 additionally expressing 11 C-terminal sequence variants of ρ-TIA (Table S5). A single ρ-TIA transcript (Tu053) was common to both the specimens, with 2 reads in S1 and 81 reads in S2 (Table S2). A mass corresponding to ρ-TIA (2389.22 Da) was detected by LC/MS at modest levels in the P, PC and DC venom duct sections of S2 (Figure 3; Figure 4), although no MS/MS fragments of ρ-TIA could be detected. In addition to ρ-TIA, a mass corresponding to T1.1 (1904.249 Da) was detected by LC/MS in the P and PC sections, while T1.2 (1953.246 Da) was detected with relatively high intensity in the distal venom duct section that was confirmed by an MS/MS match to Tu051 (Table 2) providing the first proteomic evidence for T1.1 and T1.2 (Table S4).

2.3.6. Conopressins-Conophysin [22]

Conopressin-conophysin precursors were analysed from the venom duct transcriptomes of both specimens. Mature conopressin-T was associated with 20 unique conopressin precursors in S1 and 6 unique precursors in S2, with four common (Tu057–Tu060) to both (Table S2). Of these, three precursors (Tu057–Tu059) displayed a mature conophysin sequence that was 93% similar to conophysin-G [38]. From the proteome, we identified a mass corresponding to conopressin-T (1107.567 Da) expressed in the P, PC and DC sections of the venom duct of S2 (Figure 3), with a relatively high expression (57%) in the PC sections (Figure 4). Venom expression of conopressin-T was confirmed by MS/MS.

2.3.7. Con-ikot-ikots [37]

S1 expressed 20 and S2 expressed 11 con-ikot-ikot precursors, with eight precursors (Tu061–Tu068) common to both specimens (Table S2). This class of conotoxins is associated with different signal peptide regions and remain to be assigned to a specific superfamily. In this study, most of the expressed precursors displayed the signal sequence MAMNMSMTLSTFVMVVVAAT, similar to the signal sequence of con-ikot-ikots from *C. striatus*, despite their mature peptide region being similar to con-ikot-ikots isolated from *C. geographus* [39] (Table S3). MS/MS analysis confirmed the presence of two con-ikot-ikot peptide fragments (Tu065, 11 reads; Tu068, 28 reads) in the D and DC venom duct sections of S2 (Table 2).

2.3.8. Conoporins [40]

Three conoporin precursors (Tu069–Tu071) were common between both specimens, while S1 expressed fourteen and S2 expressed five unique precursors. MS/MS detected fragments that matched to two precursors (Tu314 with 3 reads and Tu0316 with 2 reads) across the venom duct sections of S2 (Table 2).

2.3.9. Superfamily M [41]

μ-TIIIA from *C. tulipa* is a potent inhibitor of mammalian neuronal sodium channels [41]. Surprisingly, superfamily M expression levels were low in the S1 and S2 transcriptomes (1 and 3 precursors, respectively), with all precursors being identical to TIIIA (Table S1) although the μ-TIIIA mass was not detected in the proteome. One precursor (Tu072) was common to both specimens (Table S2).

2.3.10. Conoinsulin [42]

S1 had 8 conoinsulin precursors and S2 expressed 4 precursors, with only a single precursor (Tu073) common to both (Table S2). All precursors had the signal sequence MTTLFYFLLMALGLLLYVCQSSFGNQ and comprised both the A and B chains (Table S1). No mass corresponding to conoinsulins could be identified from the proteomic analysis.

2.3.11. Conkunitzins [43]

Nineteen and 3 unique conkunitzin precursors were analysed in S1 and S2, respectively, with two precursors common to both (Tu074 and Tu075). Despite low transcriptomic expression, MS/MS analysis detected fragments that matched to two conkunitzin precursors (Tu320, 2 reads and Tu075, 12 reads) in the DC and PC venom duct sections respectively (Table 2).

2.3.12. Superfamily S [44]

A single common superfamily S precursor (Tu077) that was 91% similar to G8.3 from *C. geographus* [44] was identified in S1 and S2 (5 and 7 reads, respectively). The novel precursor had the signal sequence MMSKMGAMFVLLLLFTLASSQ and a disulfide connectivity belonging to framework VIII (10 cysteine residues, -C-C-C-C-C-C-C-C-C-C-). We have named it as putative T8.1 (Table S4) since no mass corresponding to superfamily S precursors could be detected in the proteome.

2.3.13. NewGeo-1 [12]

For both specimens, five precursors were identified (Tu081–Tu086) that displayed the signal sequence MSRLFLILLVIAVITLKADAS and were devoid of cysteine residues in the mature region. S1 also had 24 additional precursors and S2 had two additional related precursors. No masses associated with this superfamily were detected in the proteome.

2.4. Intra-Clade Transcriptomic Comparison

To analyse the extent of clade-specific conotoxin expression, the transcriptomes of S1 and S2 were compared to their closest relative, *C. geographus* [12]. The transcriptomes of both species have been generated using 454 pyrosequencing platform. Remarkably, thirteen gene superfamilies, including B1, B2, A, O1, con-ikot-ikot and conopressin-conophysin, were jointly expressed within the *Gastridium* clade (Figure 5). Despite this broad overlap, no common conotoxin precursor was analysed between *C. geographus* and *C. tulipa*, with each species displaying a unique venom duct transcriptome (Figure 5b). S2 shared two superfamilies, O2 and T, with *C. geographus*, while no superfamily was exclusively common to S1 and *C. geographus*. Additionally, *C. geographus* expressed six superfamilies exclusively, including I3, J, contryphans and contulakins (Table S6). Three superfamilies, H, conoinsulins and conoporins, were found exclusively to *C. tulipa*. While no transcriptomic evidence for conoinsulins and conoporins was reported in the transcriptomic study for *C. geographus* [12], these conotoxins have previously been detected in the venom gland of *C. geographus* [42,45]. The numbers of conotoxin precursors, across the common superfamilies, were analysed to be 10-fold higher in the *C. tulipa* venom duct transcriptome.

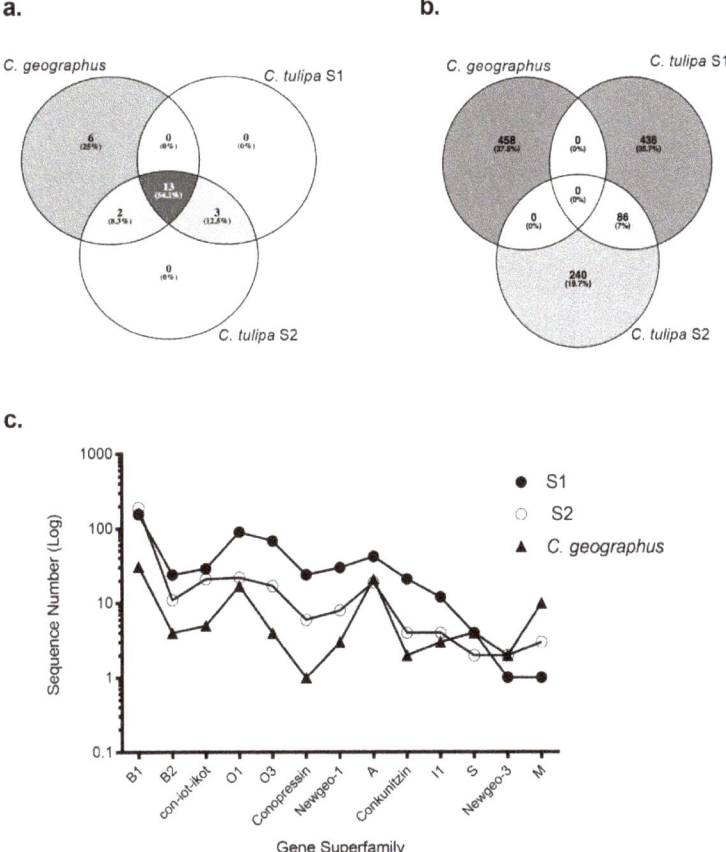

Figure 5. Intra-clade transcriptomic comparison for the *Gastridium* clade. Three-way Venn diagrams depicting the extent of the **(a)** gene superfamily and **(b)** venom duct conotoxin precursor overlap observed between *C. geographus* and *C. tulipa* (S1 and S2). Thirteen gene superfamilies were common to both the species, while six and three superfamilies were exclusive to *C. geographus* and *C. tulipa* respectively. Despite this broad overlap, both species produce a cohort of conotoxin precursors that are distinctly exclusive. **(c)** The number of conotoxin sequences expressed by both species across the 13 common gene superfamilies.

3. Discussion

Venomic studies are increasingly being used to develop comprehensive understandings of animal venoms. In this study, we describe the first venomic analysis of the piscivorous net hunter *C. tulipa* using a combination of 454 pyrosequencing, advanced mass spectrometry and dedicated bioinformatic tools. In addition, we evaluated the intra-specific mRNA variation across two *C. tulipa* specimens to better understand venom variation in Conidae. Transcriptomics uncovered 764 conotoxin precursors that were classified into 16 known superfamilies across the two specimens, with two additional superfamilies identified as unique to one specimen. Despite this superfamily overlap, 10% of the identified conotoxin precursors were found in both specimens, representing the venom 'fingerprint' for *C. tulipa*, and establishing that much of the dramatic proteomic variation previously reported [12] arises at the mRNA level [8,19,21,46–48]. Overall, the venom of *C. tulipa* is characterized by the expression of non-paralytic peptides previously hypothesized to contribute to the nirvana cabal of net hunting *Conus* species [22]. Amongst these, superfamily B1 (conantokins) was most abundant in the distal venom duct proteome, whereas conopressin-T was most abundant in the proximal venom duct, suggesting non-paralytic conotoxins may play distinct and separate roles in prey capture and/or defence in *C. tulipa*.

While geography and diet are believed to contribute to the observed venom variation between cone snail species and individuals [13,14,16], our transcriptomic comparison revealed quite distinct venom peptide repertoires despite both the specimens being collected from the same geographical region. Despite this remarkable variability, the top five gene superfamilies expressed in both *C. tulipa* specimens were B1, B2, O, A and con-ikot-ikot. Specimen S1 expressed ~ 2.5 times more conotoxin precursors than S2, with most being variants of the parent precursor. These variants were observed to be arising due to insertion/deletion of precursor sequences, an elongated post-cleavage sequence, and changes in 1-2 amino acids (in either propeptide or mature peptide); synonymous to the mRNA messiness that has been previously described [13]. For example, while the venom duct transcriptome of S2 expressed only a single variant of ρ-TIA, in S1 we analysed eleven variants of the ρ-TIA peptide (Table S5). Another contributing factor to this observed peptide variation is variable peptide processing previously identified as expanding observed conopeptide diversity [14]. These peptide variants create a diverse sequence library allowing enhanced forms to be selected in response to changing evolutionary pressures. Differences in sample preparation could also contribute to the observed intraspecific difference, with the whole venom duct retaining the epithelial cell lining [49,50] that might contribute to the increased number of peptide precursors identified in S1. Injected venom has also shown prominent intraspecific differences [19], however, we were unable to obtain injected venom from our live specimens to investigate milked venom variation in *C. tulipa*.

This study revealed that non-paralytic conotoxins dominated the transcriptome of *C. tulipa*, including conantokins, conopressins, conkunitzins, con-ikot-ikot and conoinsulins previously proposed to contribute to the nirvana cabal [51]. Conantokins dominated the distal venom duct, suggesting a role in predation [12] and potentially reflecting deployment during net hunting by *C. tulipa*. However, despite a suggested predatory role, conopressin-T dominated the proximal and proximal central venom duct sections previously shown to contribute to the defensive venom in the closely related *C. geographus* [45]. Therefore, conopressin-T may play a role in defense [12], perhaps reflecting its shift to an antagonist of the vasopressin receptor [32]. Conoinsulins have been recently implicated in the nirvana cabal of *C. geographus* [42], however, their transcriptomic expression was low and could not be detected in the proteome, suggesting these modified hormones likely play no more than a limited role in *C. tulipa* venom. ρ-TIA and the conkunitzins were also detected at moderate levels in distal venom duct sections and thus potentially contribute to the predatory strategy of *C. tulipa*. Whereas ρ-TIA injected into fish was non-lethal [27], its contribution to the nirvana cabal remains to be evaluated. Conkunitzins have been characterized to block human $K_V1.7$ [43], associated with the functioning of the β-cells of Langerhans and thus may cause hypoglycaemia and potentially synergise with conoinsulins as part of the nirvana cabal [52] but effects on fish and any synergy remains to be determined. In contrast, α-conotoxins (T1.1) and ω-conotoxins (TVIA, T6.1, T6.4) were identified in the proximal venom duct, suggesting these conotoxins contribute to a defensive strategy, while α-conotoxin T1.2 was detected in the distal venom duct, suggesting an involvement in *C. tulipa* predatory venom [12]. In addition, superfamilies O3, H and A were typically found in the distal central section. Given net feeders can also deploy a hook and line strategy to catch fish [12], it is plausible that their venom ducts have specialized sections for both predatory modes in addition to a specialized section for defence.

Comparing the transcriptomes of *C. tulipa* and *C. geographus* revealed these species had thirteen common gene superfamilies (Figure 5 and Table S6) [12], including high levels of the non-paralytic conantokins in the distal venom duct proteome. These findings support the view that cone snails belonging to the same evolutionary clade display similar venom profiles and functions that have arisen due to their overlapping predatory strategies [53]. However, both species have developed a unique venom peptide arsenal indicative of divergent evolution. This study showed that *C. tulipa* produced approximately 10-fold more conotoxin precursors than *C. geographus* reflecting the peptide expression at the time of mRNA preparation and are likely to vary across *C. tulipa* specimens. Both *C. tulipa* and especially *C. geographus* are considered dangerous to humans, with *C. geographus* implicated in numerous fatal stings [18]. *C. geographus* has a complex proximal venom duct profile dominated by ion channel modulating paralytic venom peptides [12,18]. Like *C. geographus*, we identified transcripts for superfamily A, M, O1 and O3 precursors that translate to putative paralytic α-, μ- and ω-conotoxins targeting the nicotinic acetylcholine receptors, voltage-gated sodium and calcium channels, respectively.

4. Materials and Methods

4.1. Transcriptome Analysis

4.1.1. Venom Collection, mRNA Extraction, cDNA Library, 454 Pyrosequencing and Assembly

Due to their low abundance at the collection site, we were limited to a small sample size for this study. Two adult *C. tulipa* specimens (measuring 60 mm) were collected from Lady Musgrave Island, Queensland, Australia under GBRMPA permit number G13/36201.1 and dissected on ice. The intact venom duct of Specimen 1 (S1) and stripped venom duct of Specimen 2 (S2) were treated with 1 mL TRIzol® reagent (Thermo Fisher, Scoresby, VIC, Australia), and the total RNA extracted following the manufacturer's instructions (Invitrogen, Carlsbad, CA, USA). Total RNA was further treated with an Oligotex Direct mRNA mini kit (Qiagen, Valencia, CA, USA) to extract mRNA. The extracted mRNA was sent for 454 pyrosequencing using a Roche GS FLX Titanium (Roche Diagnostics, Indianapolis, IN, USA) sequencer platform (one/eighth of a plate per sample) at the Australian Genomic Research Centre (University of Queensland, Brisbane, Australia). The corresponding contig assembly was obtained using Newbler 2.3 (Life Science, Frederick, CO, USA).

4.1.2. Conopeptide Sequence Analysis

Raw cDNA reads and the assembled contigs obtained from S1 and S2 were searched, filtered and clustered into different gene superfamilies by our in-house programme ConoSorter [54]. The precursor list was trimmed to remove sequences < 50 amino acids (most conotoxin precursors are 70–100 a.a. long), single reads, sequence containing ambiguous amino acids ("X"), redundant sequences, and those with signal peptide sequences displaying < 40% hydrophobicity. Unsorted precursors were checked with SignalP 4.0 [55] and precursors with a valid signal sequence clustered into different gene superfamilies. Propeptide regions, mature peptide cleavage sites, cysteine frameworks and likely posttranslational modifications (PTMs) were identified using the ConoPrec tool in ConoServer database [56]. Precursors that could not be classified using ConoPrec were considered as candidate novel gene superfamilies. Finally, all selected conopeptide precursors were submitted to a BLASTP search with default parameters and assessed for their similarity to known conopeptide precursors in the UniProt/BLAST database [57] and all housekeeping-related genes were removed. The minimum number of reads constituting a valid precursor sequence was set at 2.

4.1.3. Conotoxin Nomenclature

Two separate transcriptomes have been described in this study and thus we have serially numbered the common precursors first, and then continued the numbering for the unique precursors identified in each specimen. The identified common conotoxin precursors have been numbered as Tu001–Tu086. The identified unique precursors from each specimen have been numbered as Tu087–Tu522 for S1, and Tu087–Tu328 for S2. Nomenclature of putative new conotoxins precursors has followed the conventional nomenclature [58], wherein the identifying species is indicated with a capital letter, followed by numerical representation of the disulfide framework.

4.2. Proteome Analysis

4.2.1. Liquid Chromatography-Mass Spectrometry (LC-MS)

Prior to mRNA extraction, the crude venom from the venom duct sections of S2 was collected for proteomic analyses, as previously described [14]. Briefly, S2 was placed on ice before the venom duct was removed by dissection. Venom duct from S2 was dissected into four segments: proximal (P), proximal central (PC), distal central (DC) and distal (D) relative to the venom bulb. The dissected venom was collected by gently squeezing and stripping the duct segments with forceps. The collected venom samples were lyophilized and dry weight determined. 1 μg/μL of each soluble crude venom extract was subjected to top-down LC-MS on a SCIEX 5600 Triple TOF MS/MS mass spectrometer (Framingham, MA, USA) and a list of detected masses was generated, as previously described [14].

4.2.2. Enzyme Digestion

Fifty μL (1 μg/μL) protein samples were subjected to reduction and alkylation using 2% v/v iodoethanol and 0.5% v/v triethylphosphine respectively, as per Hale et al. [59]. The denatured proteins were subjected to enzymatic digestion with sequencing grade porcine trypsin (Promega, Auburn, VIC, Australia). Trypsin was activated in 40 mM NH_4HCO_3 buffer, pH 8.0 and a ratio of 1:100 (w/w) of enzyme to protein was used. Samples were incubated overnight at 37 °C and each digest was completed by heating the sample for 4 min on the lowest microwave power setting.

4.2.3. Liquid Chromatography-Electrospray Ionization Mass Spectrometry/Mass Spectrometry (LC-ESI-MS/MS)

The reduced, alkylated and enzyme-digested peptides were subjected to bottom-up tandem mass spectrometry on the SCIEX 5600 Triple TOF mass spectrometer, coupled to a Shimadzu 30 series HPLC. Information Dependent Acquisition (IDA) was performed on the samples as previously described [14]. The detected peptide fragments, including those with known PTMs were matched to the precursor sequences on the generated *C. tulipa* transcriptome database using the ProteinPilot v4.0.0 software (SCIEX, Framingham, MA, USA). The mass tolerance for precursor ions was set at 0.05 Da and 0.1 Da for the fragment ions. Peptide fragments with > 99% confidence intervals were selected as matching to the transcriptomic sequence.

4.3. Data Visualisation

The presented multi-omics data was visualised using Prism software, v7.0.0 (GraphPad, La Jolla, CA, USA). Venn diagrams were generated using Venny v2.1.0 software (Spanish National Centre for Biotechnology, Madrid, Spain). [60]

5. Conclusions

Through a combination of next generation sequencing and advanced proteomics, we have identified 764 conotoxin precursors across two specimens of *C. tulipa*. Amongst these, the dominant expression of non-paralytic peptide classes, including conantokins, conopressins and con-ikot-ikots, reaffirm their putative involvement in the net hunting predation strategy. Additionally, the possible involvement of ρ-TIA and conkunitzins in the predation-evoked venom requires further investigation in suitable prey systems to help establish their role in prey capture. Finally, through this study we have expanded our understanding of the venom profile of the *Gastridium* clade that includes two of the most lethal cone snails known to man.

Supplementary Materials: The following are available online at http://www.mdpi.com/1660-3397/17/1/71/s1, Table S1: Unique transcriptomic precursors from S1 and S2, Table S2: Common transcriptomic precursor sequences, Table S3: *C. tulipa* peptides reported in literature and their evidence from the proteome investigation, Table S4: List of the major gene superfamilies expressed in the venom duct of S1 and S2, Table S5: List of the ρ-TIA precursor variants analysed from the S1 transcriptome, Table S6: Venom duct transcriptome expression of gene superfamilies in *C. tulipa* and *C. geographus*.

Author Contributions: M.D., S.D. and R.J.L. conceived and designed the experiments; M.D., S.D. and A.J. performed the experiments; V.L. designed and operated the ConoSorter software; M.D and S.D. analysed the data; M.D., S.D., P.F.A and R.J.L wrote the manuscript.

Funding: This research was funded by an NHMRC Program grant APP1072113 (to RJL and PFA) and ARC Discovery Grants DP160103826 (to RJL., PFA and SD) and DP170104792 (to RJL and SD). MD was supported by a UQ International Postgraduate Award and RJL by an NHMRC Principal Research Fellowship.

Acknowledgments: We would like to thank Alun Jones from the IMB Proteomics Facility for MS support.

Conflicts of Interest: The authors declare no conflict of interest.

References

1. King, G.F. Venoms as a platform for human drugs: Translating toxins into therapeutics. *Expert Opin. Biol. Ther.* **2011**, *11*, 1469–1484. [CrossRef] [PubMed]

2. Casewell, N.R.; Wüster, W.; Vonk, F.J.; Harrison, R.A.; Fry, B.G. Complex cocktails: The evolutionary novelty of venoms. *Trends Ecol. Evol.* **2013**, *28*, 219–229. [CrossRef] [PubMed]

3. Cushman, D.W.; Ondetti, M.A. History of the design of captopril and related inhibitors of angiotensin converting enzyme. *Hypoertension* **1991**, *17*, 589–592. [CrossRef]

4. Bittl, J.A.; Strony, J.; Brinker, J.A.; Ahmed, W.H.; Meckel, C.R.; Chaitman, B.R.; Maraganore, J.; Deutsch, E.; Adelman, B. Treatment with bivalirudin (Hirulog) as compared with heparin during coronary angioplasty for unstable or postinfarction angina. *N. Engl. J. Med.* **1995**, *333*, 764–769. [CrossRef] [PubMed]

5. Lewis, R.J.; Dutertre, S.; Vetter, I.; Christie, M.J. Conus venom peptide pharmacology. *Pharmacol. Rev.* **2012**, *64*, 259–298. [CrossRef] [PubMed]

6. Craig, A.G.; Bandyopadhyay, P.; Olivera, B.M. Post-translationally modified neuropeptides from Conus venoms. *Eur. J. Biochem.* **1999**, *264*, 271–275. [CrossRef] [PubMed]

7. Puillandre, N.; Duda, T.; Meyer, C.; Olivera, B.M.; Bouchet, P. One, four or 100 genera? A new classification of the cone snails. *J. Mollusc Stud.* **2014**, *81*, 1–23. [CrossRef]

8. Davis, J.; Jones, A.; Lewis, R.J. Remarkable inter-and intra-species complexity of conotoxins revealed by LC/MS. *Peptides* **2009**, *30*, 1222–1227. [CrossRef]

9. Favreau, P.; Stocklin, R. Marine snail venoms: Use and trends in receptor and channel neuropharmacology. *Curr. Opin. Pharmacol.* **2009**, *9*, 594–601. [CrossRef]

10. Lewis, R.J.; Garcia, M.L. Therapeutic potential of venom peptides. *Nat. Rev. Drug Discov.* **2003**, *2*, 790–802. [CrossRef]

11. Vetter, I.; Davis, J.L.; Rash, L.D.; Anangi, R.; Mobli, M.; Alewood, P.F.; Lewis, R.J.; King, G.F. Venomics: A new paradigm for natural products-based drug discovery. *Amino Acids* **2011**, *40*, 15–28. [CrossRef] [PubMed]

12. Dutertre, S.; Jin, A.H.; Vetter, I.; Hamilton, B.; Sunagar, K.; Lavergne, V.; Dutertre, V.; Fry, B.G.; Antunes, A.; Venter, D.J.; et al. Evolution of separate predation- and defence-evoked venoms in carnivorous cone snails. *Nat. Commun.* **2014**, *5*, 3521. [CrossRef] [PubMed]

13. Jin, A.-H.; Dutertre, S.; Kaas, Q.; Lavergne, V.; Kubala, P.; Lewis, R.J.; Alewood, P.F. Transcriptomic messiness in the venom duct of *Conus miles* contributes to conotoxin diversity. *Mol. Cell. Proteom.* **2013**, *12*, 3824–3833. [CrossRef] [PubMed]

14. Dutertre, S.; Jin, A.-H.; Kaas, Q.; Jones, A.; Alewood, P.F.; Lewis, R.J. Deep venomics reveals the mechanism for expanded peptide diversity in cone snail venom. *Mol. Cell. Proteom.* **2013**, *12*, 312–329. [CrossRef]

15. Barghi, N.; Concepcion, G.P.; Olivera, B.M.; Lluisma, A.O. High conopeptide diversity in *Conus tribblei* revealed through analysis of venom duct transcriptome using two high-throughput sequencing platforms. *Mar. Biotechnol.* **2015**, *17*, 81–98. [CrossRef] [PubMed]

16. Lavergne, V.; Harliwong, I.; Jones, A.; Miller, D.; Taft, R.J.; Alewood, P.F. Optimized deep-targeted proteotranscriptomic profiling reveals unexplored Conus toxin diversity and novel cysteine frameworks. *Proc. Natl. Acad. Sci. USA* **2015**, *112*, E3782–E3791. [CrossRef] [PubMed]

17. Chang, D.; Olenzek, A.M.; Duda, T.F. Effects of geographical heterogeneity in species interactions on the evolution of venom genes. *Proc. R. Soc. Lond.* **2015**, *282*, 20141984. [CrossRef] [PubMed]

18. Dutertre, S.; Jin, A.H.; Alewood, P.F.; Lewis, R.J. Intraspecific variations in *Conus geographus* defence-evoked venom and estimation of the human lethal dose. *Toxicon* **2014**, *91*, 135–144. [CrossRef]

19. Dutertre, S.; Biass, D.; Stocklin, R.; Favreau, P. Dramatic intraspecimen variations within the injected venom of *Conus consors*: An unsuspected contribution to venom diversity. *Toxicon* **2010**, *55*, 1453–1462. [CrossRef]

20. Rivera-Ortiz, J.A.; Cano, H.; Marí, F. Intraspecies variability and conopeptide profiling of the injected venom of *Conus ermineus*. *Peptides* **2011**, *32*, 306–316. [CrossRef]

21. Abalde, S.; Tenorio, M.J.; Afonso, C.M.; Zardoya, R. Conotoxin Diversity in Chelyconus ermineus (Born, 1778) and the Convergent Origin of Piscivory in the Atlantic and Indo-Pacific Cones. *Genome Biol. Evol.* **2018**, *10*, 2643–2662. [CrossRef] [PubMed]

22. Olivera, B.M.; Cruz, L.J. Conotoxins, in retrospect. *Toxicon* **2001**, *39*, 7–14. [CrossRef]

23. Terlau, H.; Olivera, B.M. Conus venoms: A rich source of novel ion channel-targeted peptides. *Physiol. Rev.* **2004**, *84*, 41–68. [CrossRef] [PubMed]

24. Rockel, D.; Korn, W.; Kohn, A.J. *Manual of the Living Conidae Volume 1: Indo-Pacific Region*; Mal de Mer Enterprises: Hemmen, Wiesbaden, Germany, 1995; Volume 1, p. 517.

25. Tucker, J.K.; Tenorio, M.J. *Systematic Classification of Recent and Fossil Conoidean Gastropods: With Keys to the Genera of Cone Shells*; Conchbooks: Hackenheim, Germany, 2009.

26. Sharpe, I.A.; Gehrmann, J.; Loughnan, M.L.; Thomas, L.; Adams, D.A.; Atkins, A.; Palant, E.; Craik, D.J.; Adams, D.J.; Alewood, P.F.; et al. Two new classes of conopeptides inhibit the α1-adrenoceptor and noradrenaline transporter. *Nat. Neurosci.* **2001**, *4*, 902–907. [CrossRef] [PubMed]

27. Sharpe, I.A.; Thomas, L.; Loughnan, M.; Motin, L.; Palant, E.; Croker, D.E.; Alewood, D.; Chen, S.; Graham, R.M.; Alewood, P.F.; et al. Allosteric α1-adrenoreceptor antagonism by the conopeptide ρ-TIA. *J. Biol. Chem.* **2003**, *278*, 34451–34457. [CrossRef] [PubMed]

28. Ragnarsson, L.; Wang, C.-I.A.; Andersson, Å.; Fajarningsih, D.; Monks, T.; Brust, A.; Rosengren, K.J.; Lewis, R.J. Conopeptide ρ-TIA defines a new allosteric site on the extracellular surface of the α1B-adrenoceptor. *J. Biol. Chem.* **2013**, *288*, 1814–1827. [CrossRef] [PubMed]

29. Lewis, R.J.; Schroeder, C.I.; Ekberg, J.; Nielsen, K.J.; Loughnan, M.; Thomas, L.; Adams, D.A.; Drinkwater, R.; Adams, D.J.; Alewood, P.F. Isolation and structure-activity of μ-conotoxin TIIIA, a potent inhibitor of tetrodotoxin-sensitive voltage-gated sodium channels. *Mol. Pharmacol.* **2007**, *71*, 676–685. [CrossRef] [PubMed]

30. Haack, J.A.; Rivier, J.; Parks, T.N.; Mena, E.E.; Cruz, L.J.; Olivera, B.M. Conantokin-T. A gamma-carboxyglutamate containing peptide with N-methyl-d-aspartate antagonist activity. *J. Biol. Chem.* **1990**, *265*, 6025–6029. [PubMed]

31. Hill, J.M.; Atkins, A.R.; Loughnan, M.L.; Jones, A.; Adams, D.A.; Martin, R.C.; Lewis, R.J.; Craik, D.J.; Alewood, P.F. Conotoxin TVIIA, a novel peptide from the venom of *Conus tulipa* 1. Isolation, characterization and chemical synthesis. *Eur. J. Biochem.* **2000**, *267*, 4642–4648. [CrossRef]

32. Dutertre, S.; Croker, D.; Daly, N.L.; Andersson, A.; Muttenthaler, M.; Lumsden, N.G.; Craik, D.J.; Alewood, P.F.; Guillon, G.; Lewis, R.J. Conopressin-T from *Conus tulipa* reveals an antagonist switch in vasopressin-like peptides. *J. Biol. Chem.* **2008**, *283*, 7100–7108. [CrossRef]

33. Puillandre, N.; Koua, D.; Favreau, P.; Olivera, B.M.; Stocklin, R. Molecular phylogeny, classification and evolution of conopeptides. *J. Mol. Evol.* **2012**, *74*, 297–309. [CrossRef] [PubMed]

34. McIntosh, J.M.; Hasson, A.; Spira, M.E.; Gray, W.R.; Li, W.; Marsh, M.; Hillyard, D.R.; Olivera, B.M. A new family of conotoxins that blocks voltage-gated sodium channels. *J. Biol. Chem.* **1995**, *270*, 16796–16802. [CrossRef] [PubMed]

35. Zhangsun, D.; Luo, S.; Wu, Y.; Zhu, X.; Hu, Y.; Xie, L. Novel O-superfamily Conotoxins Identified by cDNA Cloning From Three Vermivorous Conus Species. *Chem. Biol. Drug Des.* **2006**, *68*, 256–265. [CrossRef] [PubMed]

36. Santos, A.D.; McIntosh, J.M.; Hillyard, D.R.; Cruz, L.J.; Olivera, B.M. The A-superfamily of conotoxins structural and functional divergence. *J. Biol. Chem.* **2004**, *279*, 17596–17606. [CrossRef] [PubMed]

37. Hu, H.; Bandyopadhyay, P.K.; Olivera, B.M.; Yandell, M. Elucidation of the molecular envenomation strategy of the cone snail *Conus geographus* through transcriptome sequencing of its venom duct. *BMC Genom.* **2012**, *13*, 284. [CrossRef] [PubMed]

38. Cruz, L.; De Santos, V.; Zafaralla, G.; Ramilo, C.; Zeikus, R.; Gray, W.; Olivera, B.M. Invertebrate vasopressin/oxytocin homologs. Characterization of peptides from *Conus geographus* and *Conus striatus* venoms. *J. Biol. Chem.* **1987**, *262*, 15821–15824. [PubMed]

39. Walker, C.S.; Jensen, S.; Ellison, M.; Matta, J.A.; Lee, W.Y.; Imperial, J.S.; Duclos, N.; Brockie, P.J.; Madsen, D.M.; Isaac, J.T.; et al. A novel *Conus* snail polypeptide causes excitotoxicity by blocking desensitization of AMPA receptors. *Curr. Biol.* **2009**, *19*, 900–908. [CrossRef] [PubMed]

40. Violette, A.; Biass, D.; Dutertre, S.; Koua, D.; Piquemal, D.; Pierrat, F.; Stocklin, R.; Favreau, P. Large-scale discovery of conopeptides and conoproteins in the injectable venom of a fish-hunting cone snail using a combined proteomic and transcriptomic approach. *J. Proteom.* **2012**, *75*, 5215–5225. [CrossRef]

41. Corpuz, G.P.; Jacobsen, R.B.; Jimenez, E.C.; Watkins, M.; Walker, C.; Colledge, C.; Garrett, J.E.; McDougal, O.; Li, W.; Gray, W.R.; et al. Definition of the M-conotoxin superfamily: Characterization of novel peptides from molluscivorous Conus venoms. *Biochemistry* **2005**, *44*, 8176–8186. [CrossRef]

42. Safavi-Hemami, H.; Gajewiak, J.; Karanth, S.; Robinson, S.D.; Ueberheide, B.; Douglass, A.D.; Schlegel, A.; Imperial, J.S.; Watkins, M.; Bandyopadhyay, P.K.; et al. Specialized insulin is used for chemical warfare by fish-hunting cone snails. *Proc. Natl. Acad. Sci. USA* **2015**, *112*, 1743–1748. [CrossRef]

43. Bayrhuber, M.; Vijayan, V.; Ferber, M.; Graf, R.; Korukottu, J.; Imperial, J.; Garrett, J.E.; Olivera, B.M.; Terlau, H.; Zweckstetter, M.; et al. Conkunitzin-S1 is the first member of a new Kunitz-type neurotoxin family. Structural and functional characterization. *J. Biol. Chem.* **2005**, *280*, 23766–23770. [CrossRef] [PubMed]

44. Liu, L.; Wu, X.; Yuan, D.; Chi, C.; Wang, C. Identification of a novel S-superfamily conotoxin from vermivorous *Conus caracteristicus*. *Toxicon* **2008**, *51*, 1331–1337. [CrossRef] [PubMed]

45. Safavi-Hemami, H.; Hu, H.; Gorasia, D.G.; Bandyopadhyay, P.K.; Veith, P.D.; Young, N.D.; Reynolds, E.C.; Yandell, M.; Olivera, B.M.; Purcell, A.W. Combined proteomic and transcriptomic interrogation of the venom gland of *Conus geographus* uncovers novel components and functional compartmentalization. *Mol. Cell. Proteom.* **2014**, *13*, mcp-M113. [CrossRef] [PubMed]

46. Rodriguez, A.M.; Dutertre, S.; Lewis, R.J.; Marí, F. Intraspecific variations in *Conus purpurascens* injected venom using LC/MALDI-TOF-MS and LC-ESI-TripleTOF-MS. *Anal. Bioanal. Chem.* **2015**, *407*, 6105–6116. [CrossRef] [PubMed]

47. Romeo, C.; Di Francesco, L.; Oliverio, M.; Palazzo, P.; Massilia, G.R.; Ascenzi, P.; Polticelli, F.; Schininà, M.E. *Conus ventricosus* venom peptides profiling by HPLC-MS: A new insight in the intraspecific variation. *J. Sep. Sci.* **2008**, *31*, 488–498. [CrossRef] [PubMed]

48. Himaya, S.; Marí, F.; Lewis, R.J. Accelerated proteomic visualization of individual predatory venoms of *Conus purpurascens* reveals separately evolved predation-evoked venom cabals. *Sci. Rep.* **2018**, *8*, 330. [CrossRef]

49. Endean, R.; Duchemin, C. The venom apparatus of Conus magus. *Toxicon* **1967**, *4*, 275–284. [CrossRef]

50. Marshall, J.; Kelley, W.P.; Rubakhin, S.S.; Bingham, J.-P.; Sweedler, J.V.; Gilly, W.F. Anatomical correlates of venom production in Conus californicus. *Biol. Bull.* **2002**, *203*, 27–41. [CrossRef]

51. Olivera, B.M.; Seger, J.; Horvath, M.P.; Fedosov, A.E. Prey-Capture Strategies of Fish-Hunting Cone Snails: Behavior, Neurobiology and Evolution. *Brain Behav. Evol.* **2015**, *86*, 58–74. [CrossRef]

52. Terlau, H.; Finol-Urdaneta, R.; Becker, S.; Raasch, W. Use of Conkunitzin-s1 for the Modulation of Glucose-Induced Insulin Secretion. U.S. Patent 13/057,809, 15 September 2011.

53. Puillandre, N.; Bouchet, P.; Duda, T.F., Jr.; Kauferstein, S.; Kohn, A.J.; Olivera, B.M.; Watkins, M.; Meyer, C. Molecular phylogeny and evolution of the cone snails (Gastropoda, Conoidea). *Mol. Phylogen. Evol.* **2014**, *78*, 290–303. [CrossRef]

54. Lavergne, V.; Dutertre, S.; Jin, A.; Lewis, R.J.; Taft, R.J.; Alewood, P.F. Systematic interrogation of the *Conus marmoreus* venom duct transcriptome with ConoSorter reveals 158 novel conotoxins and 13 new gene superfamilies. *BMC Genom.* **2013**, *14*, 708. [CrossRef] [PubMed]

55. Petersen, T.N.; Brunak, S.; von Heijne, G.; Nielsen, H. SignalP 4.0: Discriminating signal peptides from transmembrane regions. *Nat. Methods* **2011**, *8*, 785–786. [CrossRef] [PubMed]

56. Kaas, Q.; Westermann, J.C.; Craik, D.J. Conopeptide characterization and classifications: An analysis using ConoServer. *Toxicon* **2010**, *55*, 1491–1509. [CrossRef] [PubMed]

57. Altschul, S.F.; Gish, W.; Miller, W.; Myers, E.W.; Lipman, D.J. Basic local alignment search tool. *J. Mol. Biol.* **1990**, *215*, 403–410. [CrossRef]

58. King, G.F.; Gentz, M.C.; Escoubas, P.; Nicholson, G.M. A rational nomenclature for naming peptide toxins from spiders and other venomous animals. *Toxicon* **2008**, *52*, 264–276. [CrossRef] [PubMed]

59. Hale, J.E.; Butler, J.P.; Gelfanova, V.; You, J.-S.; Knierman, M.D. A simplified procedure for the reduction and alkylation of cysteine residues in proteins prior to proteolytic digestion and mass spectral analysis. *Anal. Biochem.* **2004**, *333*, 174–181. [CrossRef] [PubMed]

60. Oliveros, J.C. Venny. An Interactive Tool for Comparing Lists with Venn Diagrams. Available online: http://bioinfogp.cnb.csic.es/tools/venny/index.html (accessed on 30 November 2018).

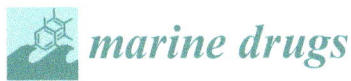

Review

Marine Toxins Targeting Kv1 Channels: Pharmacological Tools and Therapeutic Scaffolds

Rocio K. Finol-Urdaneta [1,2,*], Aleksandra Belovanovic [3,†], Milica Micic-Vicovac [3,†], Gemma K. Kinsella [4], Jeffrey R. McArthur [1] and Ahmed Al-Sabi [3,*]

[1] Illawarra Health and Medical Research Institute, University of Wollongong, Wollongong, NSW 2522, Australia; jeffreym@uow.edu.au
[2] Electrophysiology Facility for Cell Phenotyping and Drug Discovery, Wollongong, NSW 2522, Australia
[3] College of Engineering and Technology, American University of the Middle East, Kuwait; Aleksandra.B@aum.edu.kw (A.B.); Milica.Micic-vicovac@aum.edu.kw (M.M.-V.)
[4] School of Food Science and Environmental Health, College of Sciences and Health, Technological University Dublin, D07 ADY7 Dublin, Ireland; Gemma.Kinsella@tudublin.ie
* Correspondence: rfinolu@uow.edu.au (R.K.F.-U.); Ahmed.Al-Sabi@aum.edu.kw (A.A.-S.); Tel.: +965-22251400 (ext.1798) (A.A.-S.)
† These authors contributed equally to this review.

Received: 3 February 2020; Accepted: 16 March 2020; Published: 20 March 2020

Abstract: Toxins from marine animals provide molecular tools for the study of many ion channels, including mammalian voltage-gated potassium channels of the Kv1 family. Selectivity profiling and molecular investigation of these toxins have contributed to the development of novel drug leads with therapeutic potential for the treatment of ion channel-related diseases or channelopathies. Here, we review specific peptide and small-molecule marine toxins modulating Kv1 channels and thus cover recent findings of bioactives found in the venoms of marine Gastropod (cone snails), Cnidarian (sea anemones), and small compounds from cyanobacteria. Furthermore, we discuss pivotal advancements at exploiting the interaction of κM-conotoxin RIIIJ and heteromeric Kv1.1/1.2 channels as prevalent neuronal Kv complex. RIIIJ's exquisite Kv1 subtype selectivity underpins a novel and facile functional classification of large-diameter dorsal root ganglion neurons. The vast potential of marine toxins warrants further collaborative efforts and high-throughput approaches aimed at the discovery and profiling of Kv1-targeted bioactives, which will greatly accelerate the development of a thorough molecular toolbox and much-needed therapeutics.

Keywords: bioactives; conotoxins 2; Kv1; marine toxins; modulators; potassium channels; sea anemone toxins

1. Introduction

1.1. Kv1 Channels

Voltage-gated K$^+$ channels (Kv) are intrinsic plasma membrane proteins mediating the selective flow of K$^+$ ions down their electrochemical gradient in response to a depolarization in the transmembrane electric field [1]. The selectivity and voltage dependence of Kv channels make them central players in virtually all physiological functions, including the maintenance and modulation of neuronal [2–4] and muscular (both cardiac and skeletal) excitability [5–7], regulation of calcium signalling cascades (reviewed by Reference [8]), control of cell volume [9,10], immune response [11], hormonal secretion [12], and others.

The Kv channel α-subunit belongs to the six transmembrane (6-TM) family of ion channels (Figure 1a,b) in which the voltage-sensing domain (VSD) formed by transmembrane segments S1–S4 controls pore opening via the S4–S5 intracellular loop that is connected to the pore domain (PD).

The PD is formed by transmembrane segments S5–S6 including a re-entrant pore loop bearing the potassium selectivity sequence TVGYG [13]. Depolarization of the transmembrane electric field induces a conformational change in the VSD that leads to channel *activation*, leading to opening of the water-filled permeation pathway permitting K^+ to flow down their electrochemical gradient. Upon repolarization, the VSD returns to its resting state, closing the channel gate and terminating ionic flow in a process called deactivation. Immediately after deactivation, channels can be reactivated; however, if depolarization-induced channel activation extends beyond a few milliseconds, inactivation ensues, ceasing K^+ permeability. Kv channels recover from inactivation only after spending enough time at a hyperpolarized potential [14]. The molecular underpinnings of the inactivation processes have been thoroughly examined functionally and structurally, identifying various inactivation types involving distinct and complex molecular mechanisms. Voltage-gated ion channels can inactivate from pre-open closed-states (closed-state inactivation, CSI) or from the open state(s) (open-state inactivation, OSI) [15]. Inactivation can also be categorized depending on the speed of its onset upon activation. In some Kv channels, fast inactivation or N-type inactivation occurs soon after the channel activates and it is mainly due to an intracellular block by the channel's intracellular N-terminus hence known as the inactivation particle [16]. This process has been directly observed by cryo-electron microscopy (cryo-EM) in a related prokaryotic K channel [17]. In addition to N-type inactivation, a common but relatively slower process happens after tens or hundreds of milliseconds from channel activation that is termed C-type (or slow) inactivation [18]. Even though the extent and complexity of slow inactivation remain the subjects of investigation, the pore structure and the permeating ions appear to play a vital role [19]. Recent structural and functional studies support a mechanism through which the redistribution of structural water molecules accompanies the rearrangement of amino acids within the channel's inner cavity and outer vestibule, ultimately leading to the collapse of the permeation pathway in C-type inactivation (reviewed in Reference [20]). Modulation of the inactivation process is a powerful strategy to control the cellular availability of Kv channel-mediated currents; thus, both N- and C-type inactivation are responsive to the cellular redox environment [21]. For instance, structural motifs within the Kv channel's N-terminus/inactivation particle serve as sensors of the cytoplasmic redox potential [22].

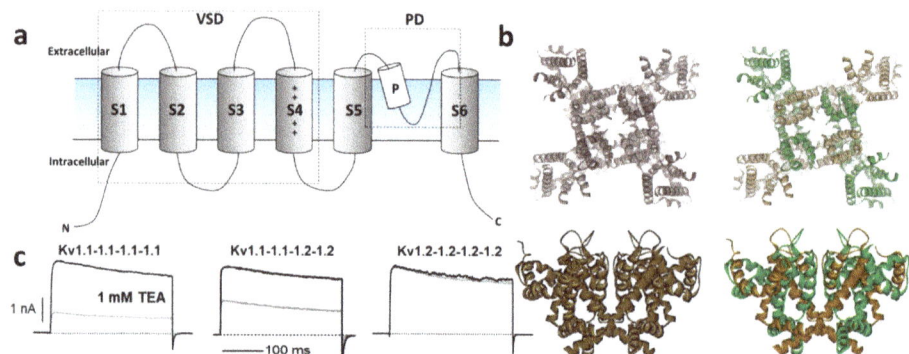

Figure 1. (**a**) Schematic illustration of K_V channel membrane topology depicting the 6 transmembrane subunits including the voltage sensing domain (voltage-sensing domain (VSD): S1–S4) and the pore domain (PD) between S5 and S6 segments. (**b**) Top and side views of representative homomeric and heteromeric Kv1 channels based on the crystal structure of Kv1.2 channels [(Protein Data Bank number, PDB: 2A79)] [13]. (**c**) Current trances of homomeric Kv1.1 (left) and 1.2 (right) channels and their heteromeric combination (middle) revealing distinct sensitivity to the classical pharmacological tool tetraethylammonium (TEA) [23,24].

K$^+$ channels are the most diverse family of ion channels in excitable and nonexcitable tissues, encompassing 40 Kv members allocated into 12 subfamilies: voltage-gated Kv subfamilies, the *Ether-à-go go* (EAG) subfamily, and the Ca^{2+}-activated subfamilies [1]. As such, they are implicated in many neurological, cardiac, and autoimmune disorders, which position them as important therapeutic targets [25]. The identified genes for Kv channel α-subunits are classified into twelve subfamilies: Kv1 (Shaker); Kv2 (Shab); Kv3 (Shaw); Kv4 (Shal); Kv7 (KvLQT); Kv10 (HERG); Kv11 (EAG); Kv12 (ELK); and the modulatory "electrically silent" Kv5, Kv6, Kv8, and Kv9 subfamilies (https://doi.org/10.2218/gtopdb/F81/2019.4). The *Shaker*-related Kv1 family is comprised of eight members (Kv1.1–Kv1.8) encoded by the corresponding *KCNA1–KCNA8* genes. Several Kv1 channels have been identified and functionally characterized within their native tissues, exploiting selective blockers (reviewed by References [2,26,27]). The first Kv1 complexes were purified from mammalian brain using the snake venom toxins called dendrotoxins (DTX). These studies indicated that the functional Kv1 channel is a large (Mr ~400 kDa) sialoglycoprotein complex consisting of four pore-forming α-subunits and four cytoplasmically associated auxiliary β-proteins [28] that modulate K$^+$ channel activation and inactivation kinetics (for a thorough review, refer to Reference [29]).

The Kv1 channels are expressed in a variety of tissues as homo- or heterotetrameric complexes (Figure 1a,b) [30]. These complexes are formed in the endoplasmic reticulum [31], where monomers are randomly recruited, assembled, and inserted in the plasma membrane [31]. The four cytoplasmic N-terminal domains interact with one another in a strictly subfamily-specific manner, thus providing the molecular basis for the selective formation of heteromultimeric channels in vivo [32,33]. The predominant pathway in tetramer formation involves dimerization of subunit dimers, thereby creating interaction sites different from those involved in the monomer–monomer association during the oligomerization process [34].

In heterologous expression systems, all Potassium Voltage-gated channel subfamily A Member gene (*KCNA*) transcripts encoding Kv1 α-subunits yield functional homo-tetrameric complexes with distinct biophysical and pharmacological profiles [35], (Figure 1c). While theoretically, the combination of different Kv1 subunits could afford impressive functional diversity, only a subset of oligomeric combinations has been elucidated [36–40], suggesting their synthesis and/or assembly are carefully orchestrated. Amongst the K$_V$1 channels, Kv1.2 is the most prevalent isoform in neuronal membranes where only a small fraction occurs as a homo-tetramer, while the majority are a hetero-tetramer with other Kv1 α-subunits [36,10]. In these preparations, the less abundant Kv1.1 subunit is consistently identified in oligomers containing Kv1.2 channels.

1.2. Mechanisms of Kv Channel Inhibition by Marine Toxins

The diversity of Kv1 channels and their wide distribution, including their specific expression pattern in the central and peripheral nervous systems (CNS and PNS, respectively), together with their vital function in the excitability of nerve and muscle, make them strategic targets of marine toxins. These natural products are synthesized by marine organisms to deter competitors and to aid predation or for self-defense [41]. Many venomous organisms block Kv channel-mediated currents, crippling membrane repolarization, yielding enhanced excitability, and ultimately engendering paralysis in pray or foe [42].

Marine toxins exploit different Kv channel traits to exert their modulatory actions. A commonly used strategy relies on direct occlusion of the narrow potassium permeation pathway from the extracellular side of the channel protein (Figure 2a,b). Toxins inhibiting ionic current via this mechanism are referred to as "pore blockers". Many structurally and phylogenetically unrelated pore-blocking toxins of Kv channels share a dyad motif composed of a lysine (positive) and a tyrosine/phenylalanine (hydrophobic) [43–45]. The lysine residue fits snugly in the Kv channel selectivity filter, sterically occluding K$^+$ ion flow, whilst the hydrophobic amino acid in the dyad aids docking and consolidation of the toxin binding. This dyad motif has been proposed to be the minimal core domain of the Kv channel-binding pharmacophore (Figure 2b) [46–49].

Mutational analysis and docking calculations have demonstrated that some marine toxins do not possess the canonical functional dyad or do not seem to use one in the classic "pore blocker" fashion to prevent potassium permeation. In these toxins, a positively charged ring of amino acids participates in electrostatic interactions with the Kv1 outer vestibule. These residues provide surface recognition and anchoring, and concurrently, a network of hydrogen bonds and hydrophobic interactions consolidate "capping" of the channel vestibule, with the peptide toxin acting as a lid over the Kv channel pore (Figure 2b) [50].

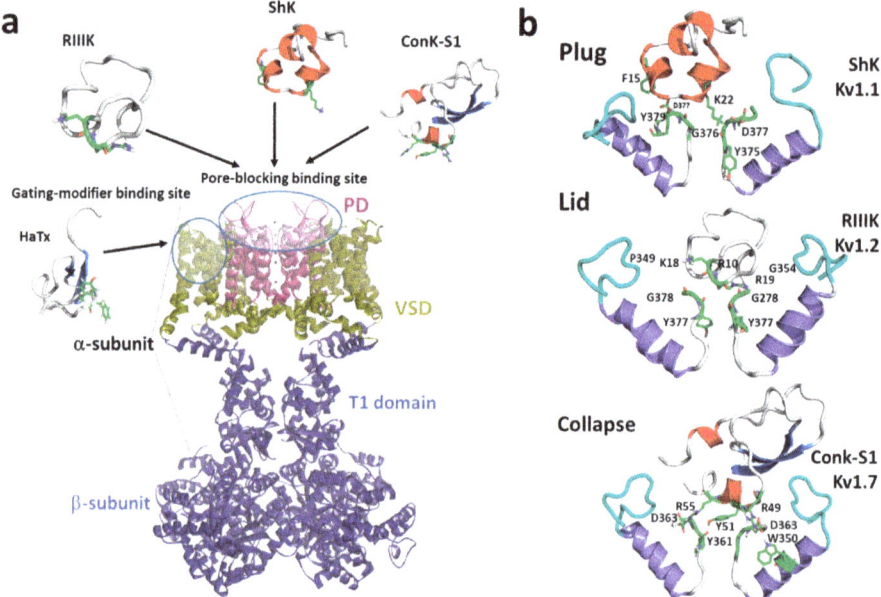

Figure 2. (**a**) Schematic presentation of a side view K$_V$1 channel showing the site of interaction with representative pore-blocking peptide toxins from Cone snail (κM-RIIIK, [51] and ConK-S1, PDB: 2CA7, [52]) and sea anemone ShK (PDB: 1ROO, [53]) and gating modifier toxin from spider (HaTx; PDB: 1D1H, [54]). (**b**) The modes of pore blocking (plug, lid, or collapse) illustrated by marine peptide blockers as revealed by the docking models. The outer turret regions (residues 348–359 for Kv1.1, 350–359 for Kv1.2, and 334–343 for Kv1.7) are in cyan, and the inner turret regions (residues 377–386 for Kv1.1, 377–386 for Kv1.2, and 462–469 for Kv1.7) are indicated in green. Only two subunits of the Kv1 channels are shown, for simplicity. Docking was performed using the Haddock webserver [55,56] and the docking model image were generated using Pymol (The PyMOL Molecular Graphics System, [57]).

A distinct mechanism from pore block is achieved by interacting with the gating mechanism of Kv channels. Toxins acting in this fashion are known as "gating modifiers". The VSD in Kv channels controls pore opening; hence, toxins binding to the extracellularly exposed linker between transmembrane segments S3 and S4, the S3–S4 linker paddle motif within the VSD, inhibit channel function by increasing the energy required to open the channel's gate by shifting the voltage dependence of activation to more depolarized potentials. Alternatively, some toxins destabilize the Kv channel open state reflected as enhanced entry into a nonconductive inactivated state at potentials where Kv activity would normally be favored [58]. This modulatory mechanism was first shown for Hanatoxin, a gating modifier peptide component of the Chilean rose-hair tarantula venom that inhibits Kv2.1 channels (Figure 2a) [59].

A recently proposed inhibitory mechanism appears as a hybrid strategy between pore blockade and gating modification. A toxin sitting in the channel's outer vestibule blocks the extracellular side of the permeation pathway and modifies the permeation of water molecules into proteinaceous peripheral cavities in the channel. This creates asymmetries in the distribution of water molecules around the selectivity filter, triggering a local collapse of the channel pore akin to Kv C-type inactivation (Figure 2b) [60].

2. Molluscan Peptides that Inhibit Kv1 Channels

Conotoxins constitute a family of small peptide toxins found in the venom glands of cone snails [61]. These marine gastropods of the genus *Conus* are represented by ~800 predatory mollusks [62]. It is believed that the large arsenal of conotoxins within a single venom is used for fast pray immobilization in hunting cone snails [63].

Conotoxins are typically 8–60 amino acid peptides that potently interact with a wide range of voltage- and ligand-gated ion channels and receptors [64]. The cone snail venom peptides evolved to capture their prey (worms, fish, and other mollusks), and their venom is known to interact and modulate several mammalian ion channels with great selectivity [65]. The pharmacological properties of conotoxins have been exploited as molecular tools for the study of mammalian targets [66], and their scaffolds are employed for drug development and potential treatment of human diseases [67].

Mature conotoxins are structurally diverse, including disulfide-free and mono- and poly-disulfide-bonded peptides (several reviews deal with the structural diversity of conotoxins; see References [64,68]). Peptides lacking disulfide bonds are flexible, whereas the presence of multiple disulfide linkages provides structural rigidity and provides different three-dimensional conformations depending on the cysteine disulfide framework within the toxin sequence [69]. Cone snail VDPs are often post-translationally modified, including C-terminal amidation, bromination, γ-carboxylation, hydroxylation, O-glycosylation, N-terminal pyroglutamylation, and sulfation [70].

Pharmacological classification of the structurally diverse (i.e., cysteine framework/connectivity, loop length, and fold) conotoxins is based on the target type and mechanism of action of the peptides. Twelve pharmacological families are currently recognized (ConoServer [71]). Due to the variable nature of conotoxins, a consensus classification-linking pharmacology to structure has not been agreed upon. Given the nature of this review, we will focus on the pharmacological family classification of the kappa- or κ-conotoxins, which are defined by modulatory activity over potassium-selective channels. The founding member of the κ-conotoxins was identified in the venom of the piscivorous snail *Conus purpurascens* κ-PVIIA by its potent block of *Drosophila* voltage-gated *Shaker* channels [72].

Up to now, nine conotoxins are listed as mammalian Kv1 channel blockers in the Kalium database [73]. From those, the activity of Contryphan-Vn from *Conus ventricosus* against Kv1.1 and Kv1.2 was tested by displacement of radiolabeled *Bunodosoma granulifera* Kv1 blocker (BgK), showing weak activity at 600 μM [74]. Therefore, Contryphan-Vn modulatory activity against Kv1 channels remains to be verified.

The other κ-conotoxins listed belong to various structural families of disulfide-rich peptides (A, I, J, M, O, and the Conkunitzins; Figure 3 and Table 1). Disulfide-rich κ-conotoxins have been shown to act as pore blockers using canonical interactions through the "functional dyad" and the "ring of basic residues" as molecular determinants of κ-conotoxin modulation of Kv1 channel conductance. Such mechanisms of action have been described in scorpion and cnidarian VDP toxins blocking Kv1 channels; hence, κ-conotoxins share important features that enable Kv1 channel inhibition in a similar way to other animal VDP blockers.

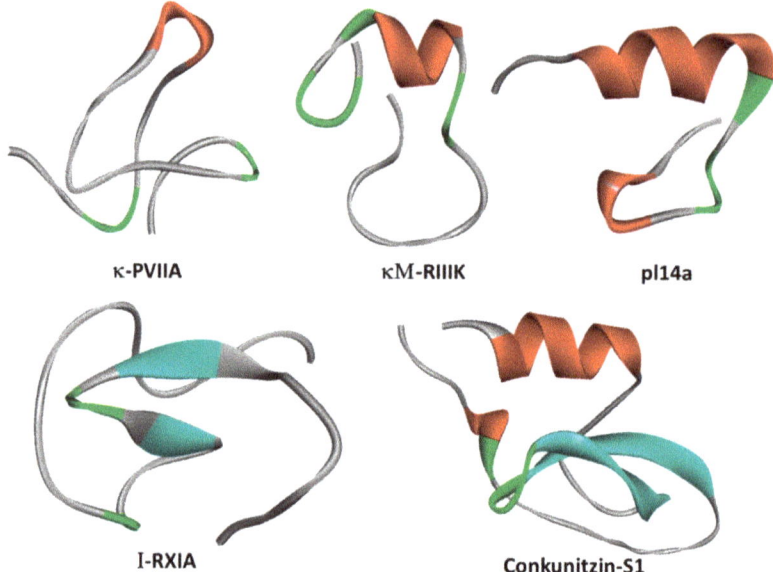

Figure 3. Structures of representative cone snail venom-derived peptide toxins κ-PVIIA (PDB: 1AV3, [75]), κM-RIIIK [51], pl14a (PDB: 2FQC, [76]), I-RXIA (PDB: 2JTU, http://www.rcsb.org/structure/2JTU), and Conkunitzin-S1 (PDB: 2CA7, [52]): β-sheets are in cyan, and α-helices are in red.2.1. κM-RIIIK.

Despite the great abundance of *Conus* peptides characterized to date, relatively few have been shown to interact with Kv channels. κM-RIIIK from *Conus radiatus* [77] (Figures 2 and 3) is 24 residues long, and it is structurally homologous to the well-known voltage-gated sodium channel blocker μ-GIIIA [78]. RIIIK was originally identified as a Shaker (*Drosophila*) and TSha1 (trout) Kv1 orthologue channel blocker [79]. Later, RIIIK became the first conotoxin described to modulate human Kv1 channels, selectively blocking homomeric Kv1.2 without apparent effects over Navs or mammalian homologs Kv1.1, Kv1.3, Kv1.4, Kv1.5, and Kv1.6 recorded by Two Electrode Voltage Clamp recording (TEVC) in *Xenopus* oocytes [77]. Interestingly, heteromerization with Kv1.2 α-subunits suffices to render Kv1.1, Kv1.5, and Kv1.7, containing heterodimeric channels sensitive to low micromolar RIIIK [80].

Binding of κM-RIIIK to closed (deactivated) Kv1.2 channels is ~2-fold stronger than to the open state, hinting towards state-dependent interactions between this peptide and the Kv1s. Importantly, RIIIK blocks its Kv1 channel targets, through a pharmacophore comprised of a ring of positive charges and not via the classical "dyad motif" [51,81].

2.1. κM-RIIIJ

Further analyses of the venom of *Conus radiatus* revealed a second, closely related peptide, named κM-RIIIJ, that displayed 10-fold higher potency (~30 nM) blocking homomeric Kv1.2-mediated currents. Comparison of RIIIK and RIIIJ activity in an animal model of ischemia/reperfusion revealed that the latter was cardioprotective, an effect adjudicated to RIIIJ's higher potency at inhibiting heterodimeric Kv1-mediated currents [80].

An in-depth evaluation of RIIIJ was performed against heteromeric channels generated by a covalent linkage composed of Kv1.2 and all other Kv1s subunits (except for Kv1.8) at different stoichiometries and arrangements [82]. This work revealed that RIIIJ exquisitely targets asymmetric Kv channels composed of three Kv1.2 subunits and one Kv1.1 or Kv1.6 subunit. RIIIJ's apparent affinity for the asymmetric complex is ~100-fold higher than for the homomeric Kv1.2 complex.

Recently, the discerning sensitivity of RIIIJ to its heteromeric Kv1 channel target was exploited to comprehensively classify and characterize individual somatosensory neuronal subclasses within heterogenous populations of dorsal root ganglion (DRG) neurons [83]. RIIIJ's selectivity was used to distinguish two functional Kv1 complexes in mouse dorsal root ganglion (DRG) neurons. One being RIIIJ's high-affinity target ($3 \times$ Kv1.2 + Kv1.1 or Kv1.6), and the second component characterized by inhibition at higher RIIIJ concentrations arguably composed of homo-tetrameric Kv1.2 subunits [82]. The functional behavior of large DRG (L-DRG) neurons exposed to RIIIJ was used to classify L-DRGs in six discrete neuronal subpopulations (L1–L6). Interestingly, this peptide's block of heteromeric Kv1 channels in subclass L3 and L5 neurons lead to enhanced calcium signals consistent with their contribution to repolarization after a depolarizing stimulus, whilst in subclass L1 and L2 neurons, exposure to RIIIJ decreased the threshold for action potential firing. The integration of constellation pharmacology [66], electrophysiology, and transcriptomic profiling using RIIIJ as a pharmacological tool served to functionally assess three biological levels spanning the molecular target Kv1 channel (Kv1.2/Kv1.1 heteromer), the functional characteristics of specific neuronal subclasses and the physiological system (i.e., proprioception) in which they participate.

Table 1. Some characteristics of known conotoxins targeting the Kv1 channel.

Conopeptide	Source	Family	Target Channel(s) (IC$_{50}$)	References
CPY-Pl1	*C. planorbis*	CPY	Kv1.2 (2 µM); Kv1.6 (170 nM)	[84]
CPY-Fe1	*C. ferruginesus*	CPY	Kv1.2 (30 µM); Kv1.6 (8.8 µM)	[84]
κM-RIIIJ	*C. radiatus*	M	hKv1.2 (33 nM)	[80]
κM-RIIIK	*C. radiatus*	M	hKv1.2 (300 nM) rKv1.2 (335 nM)	[79]
Pl14a (κJ-PlXIVA)	*C. planorbis*	J	hKv1.6 (1.6 µM)	[76]
κ-ViTx	*C. vigro*	I2	rKv1.1 (1.6 µM) rKv1.3	[85]
Conkunitzin-S1	*C. Striatus*	Conkunitzins	Kv1.7 (< nM)	[12]

2.2. Conk-S1

Conk-S1 (Conkunitzin-S1; Figures 2 and 3) was the first reported member of a novel family of marine toxins characterized by the Kunitz structural fold [52]. Conk-S1 is a 60-residue marine toxin from the venom of *Conus striatus* that blocks Shaker [52] and mammalian Kv1 channels [12]. The crystal structure of Conk-S1 displays a Kunitz-type fold in which an NH$_2$- terminal 3-10 helix, 2-stranded β-sheet, and the COOH- terminal α-helix are stabilized by 2 disulfide bridges and a network of non-covalent interactions [86]. Despite having only two of the three highly conserved cysteine bridges present in canonical Kunitz peptides, such as bovine pancreatic trypsin inhibitor (BPTI) and Dendrotoxin-κ, structural analyses using NMR spectroscopy verified the presence of the Kunitz-type fold not only in Conk-S1 but also in its homolog Conk-S2 [87].

A comprehensive selectivity profile amongst Kv1, Kv2, Kv3, Kv4, BK and EAG channels is available for Conk-S1 [12]. With such information in hand, it was possible to utilize Conk-S1 as a pharmacological tool to identify the role of Kv1.7 channels in glucose-stimulated insulin secretion (GSIS) in pancreatic β cells [12]. Conk-S1 not only was useful as a molecular tool but also was shown to enhance insulin secretion ex vivo in a glucose-dependent manner in islets of Langerhans as well as in vivo in anesthetized rats. Rats treated with Conk-S1 did not evidence any adverse effects, highlighting the potential of Conk-S1 as a therapeutic scaffold for the treatment of hyperglycemia related disorders.

Mutation of the *Shaker* K$^+$ channel residue K427 to aspartate enhances Conk-S1 potency of block >2000-fold, suggesting Conk-S1 interactions with the Kv channel vestibule (see Figure 2b) [52]. Recent structural, functional, and computational work proposes a novel mechanism of the block for K$^+$ channel blockers [60]. Conk-S1 does not seem to directly block the ion conduction pathway, but instead, its binding causes disruptions in the structural water network responsible for the stabilization of the Kv channel activated state [88], causing the collapse of the permeation and the consequent hindrance of K^+ ion flow, similar to what has been described to occur during slow inactivation [60]. This systematic and elegant work was performed on Kv1.2 channels (Conk-S1, IC_{50}: 3.4 ± 1.3 μM) instead of the previously described highest affinity mammalian target Kv1.7. The affinity of Conk-S1 for human Kv1.7 channels is 37 ± 5 nM (*Xenopus* oocytes [89]) and 439 ± 82 nM for the mouse orthologue determined in mammalian cells [12]. Interestingly, comparison of the pore sequences of Kv1.1–Kv1.6 and Shaker channels lead to the conclusion that Conk-S1's preferential toxin action against the Drosophila channel (502 ± 140 nM, *Xenopus* oocytes) was dominated by aromatic interactions mediated by a phenylalanine in Shaker position 425, whilst in hKv1.7, a histidine (341) is present in the equivalent position.

The observation that heteromerization with Kv1.7 enhances Conk-S1 affinity towards Kv1.2 containing hetero-multimeric Kv channels [12] suggests that such a mechanism of block would extend to Kv1.7-mediated current inhibition as well as to other homo and hetero-tetrameric Kv1 channels.

2.3. κ-PVIIA

The venom of *Conus purpurascens* is a source of the founding member of the kappa conotoxins κ-PVIIA (or CGX-1051). PVIIA is a 27-amino-acid-long peptide that potently blocks Shaker potassium channels [72,75]. PVIIA was reported to reduce myocardial lesions in rabbit, rats, and dogs, exhibiting protective effects relevant to ischemia/reperfusion-induced cardiomyocyte damage [90]. In these animal models, acute intravenous administration of PVIIA substantially reduces myocardium infarct size without adverse alterations in cardiovascular hemodynamics [91]. However, attempts to identify a mammalian target of PVIIA have been unsuccessful with 2 μM PVIIA failing to inhibit Kv1.1 or Kv1.4-mediated currents expressed in *Xenopus laevis* oocytes and recorded by two-electrode voltage clamp [92].

While the mechanism underlying the cardioprotective efficacy of κ-PVIIA is unclear, the reported preclinical results in animal models of ischemia/reperfusion suggest that κ-PVIIA may represent a valuable adjunct therapy in the management of acute myocardial infarction [93].

2.4. κ-ViTx

The structural superfamily I2 of *Conus* peptides was established with the discovery of κ-conotoxin ViTx in the venom of *Conus virgo*. In ViTx, four disulfide bridges crosslink a chain of 35 amino acids. TEVC recordings in *Xenopus* oocytes showed that ViTx inhibits voltage-gated K^+ channels rKv1.1 (IC_{50}: 1.59 ± 0.14 μM) and hKv1.3 (IC_{50}: 2.09 ± 0.11 μM) but not Kv1.2 (up to 4 μM). Activity on other Kv1 channels has not been reported [85].

2.5. SrXIa

SrXIa was purified from the venom of vermivorous *Conus spurius* and was found to inhibit Kv1.2 and Kv1.6 without apparent effects over Kv1.3 channels. SrXIa does not contain lysine residues and thus is considered to lack a functional dyad to support Kv1 channel blockade. Moreover, a ring of arginine including R17 and R29 were shown to be important for its biological activity [94]. Activity on other Kv1 channels is missing.

2.6. Promiscuous Conotoxins Interacting with Kv1 Channels

2.6.1. pl14a

The J-conotoxin pI14a isolated from the vermivorous cone snail *Conus planorbis* is 25 amino acids long, from which six residues form an elongated NH_2- terminus and four cysteines are bonded into the "1-3, 2-4" connectivity, and is decorated with a C-terminal amide group (Figure 3). NMR structure determination revealed one α-helix and two $3^{(10)}$-helices stabilized by two disulfide bridges [76]. pl14a inhibits Kv1.6 channels ($IC_{50} = 1.59$ μM) as well as neuromuscular α1β1εδ and neuronal α3β4 nicotinic acetylcholine receptors (IC$_{50}$s = 0.54 µM and 8.7 µM, respectively). Importantly, 1-5 µM pl14a had negligible effects over Kv1.1–Kv1.5, Kv2.1, Kv3.4, Nav1.2, or N-type presynaptic Cav channels [76]. An interesting feature of pl14a is that it contains a putative Kv channel blocking "dyad" formed by residues K18 and T19 as well as a ring of basic residues consisting of R3, R5, R12, and R25. In silico predictions suggest that pI14a inhibition of Kv1.6-mediated currents is mainly supported by the basic ring of amino acids [95]; however, this awaits experimental verification.

2.6.2. Tyrosine-Rich Conopeptides CPY-Pl1 and CPY-Fe1

The conopeptide family Y (CPY) was defined by the discovery of two 30-amino-acid-long peptides, named CPY-Pl1 and CPY-Fe1, found in the venoms of vermivorous marine snails *Conus planorbis* and *Conus ferrugineus*. VDPs belonging to this family do not contain disulfide bridges and appear unstructured in solution. Nevertheless, the NMR analysis of CPY-PI1 revealed a helical region around residues 12–18 [84].

Functionally, both peptides are more active against Kv1.6 and Kv1.2 than Kv1.1, Kv1.3, Kv1.4, and Kv1.5, with CPY-PI1 displaying ~50-fold more potency against Kv1.6 than CPY-Fe1 (IC$_{50}$ 0.17 µM and 8.8 µM, respectively), being ~18-fold more potent for pl14a. At 1 µM, these peptides also inhibit currents mediated by N-methyl-D-Aspartate (NMDA) receptors (NR1–3b/NR2A and NR1–3b/NR2B) and Nav1.2 channels. Anecdotally, devitellinized oocytes exposed to hydrophobic CPY peptides become "leaky", suggesting that these peptides could intercalate into the plasma membrane either to destabilize it or to perhaps display pore-forming activity [84].

2.6.3. µ-PIIIA

Conotoxin µ-PIIIA and µ-SIIIA inhibit mammalian Nav1.2 and Nav1.7 channels with nanomolar potency [96] and bacterial sodium channels NaChBac and NavSp1 in the picomolar range [97]. It has been recently shown that these µ-conopeptides can also selectively inhibit Kv1.1 and Kv1.6 channels with nanomolar affinity while sparing other Kv1 and Kv2 family members [96]. Functional evaluation of chimeras between µ-PIIIA sensitive and insensitive isoforms revealed that these toxins interact with the Kv pore region with subtype specificity largely determined by the extracellular loop connecting the channel pore and transmembrane helix S5 (turret).

In contrast to all other pore-blocking κ-conotoxins, the binding of µ-PIIIA to Kv1.6 channels reaches equilibrium after several tens of minutes, pointing towards an alternative Kv1 mechanism of inhibition for µ-PIIIA. Docking and molecular dynamics simulations were used to assess the interaction between µ-conotoxins and Kv1 channels [98]. This work proposed similar binding modes of µ-PIIIA to Kv1.6 and Kv1.1 homomeric channels supported by hydrogen bonding between R and K residues from µ-PIIIA's α-helical core and the central pore residues of the Kv channel. In such circumstances, effective pore blockage would occur by dual interaction of the µ-conotoxin with both inner and outer pore loops of the Kv channel. This implies that the composition of the channel inner pore loop determines the orientation of the µ-PIIIA, which is further consolidated by hydrogen bonding with the Kv1 extracellular pore loops. The subtype specificity of µ-PIIIA among the Kv1 family members was then rationalized by unfavorable electrostatic interactions between charged residues in the pore loops of the µ-PIIIA-resistant Kv1s.

The apparent binding kinetics of µ-PIIIA to Kv1.6 channels were too slow to allow estimation of potency from concertation response curves as it is customary for potassium channels blocking peptides. This poses the question of whether common peptide screenings on Kv channels performed by relatively short (~5 min) exposures to the toxins are consistently missing positive hits. Alternatively, binding equilibrium determinations in experiments that extend over tens of minutes may be providing an overestimation of potency due to intrinsic confounding factors (such as current rundown and cell viability) inherent to the biological system and experimental conditions used.

2.6.4. κP-Crassipeptides

From Crassispirine snails, a group of venomous marine gastropods, κP-crassipeptides were isolated [99]. Three peptides were characterized to be Kv1 channel blockers, CceIXa, CceIXb, and IqiIXa. The same study showed that, among the tested neuronal hKv1 channels, CceIXb was selective for Kv1.1 with IC$_{50}$ ~ 3 μM. In 1 mM concentration, the other two toxins did not elicit any detectable effects when tested on these Kv1 targets [99]. However, CceIXa and b peptides elicited an excitatory phenotype in a subset of small-diameter capsaicin-sensitive mouse DRG neurons that were affected by the Kv1.6 blocker κJ conotoxin pl14a [94,99]. Since κJ conotoxin pl14a is broader in selectivity among Kv1 channels expressed in DRGs, CceIXa might be more selective for particular combinations of heteromeric Kv1 channels.

3. Cnidarian Peptides that Inhibit Kv1 Channels

Sea anemones (phylum Cnidarian) produce various classes of peptide toxins targeting a diverse array of ion channels that serve the functions of defense from predators and immobilization of potential prey [100]. Some marine toxins found in sea anemones target Kv1 channels in which block leads to neuronal hyperexcitability and muscle spasms. These marine toxins have been shown to have important therapeutic applications in the treatment of autoimmune diseases including multiple sclerosis, rheumatoid arthritis, and diabetes [101,102].

Due to the large diversity of toxins produced from sea anemones and both their functional convergence and promiscuity, classification of sea anemone toxins has proven difficult. A recent review has attempted to circumvent this by classifying sea anemone proteinaceous toxins into three major groups: (1) enzymes, (2) nonenzymatic cytotoxins, or (3) nonenzymatic peptide neurotoxins [103]. The Kv channel targeting sea anemone toxins all fall into the third group, peptide neurotoxins, which can be further classified into 9 structural families. To date, of these subfamilies, only six have a Kv-selective toxin representative (ShK, Kv type 1; Kunitz-Domain, Kv type 2; B-Defensin-like, Kv type 3; Boundless β-hairpin (BBH), Kv type 4; Inhibitor Cystine-Knot (ICK), Kv type 5; and Proline-hinged asymmetric β-hairpin (PHAB), Kv type 6; see Table 2).

The anemone VDP toxins interact with Kv1 channels, are typically 17–66 amino acids long, and are cross-linked by 2–4 disulfide bridges [104,105]. Up to 21 sea anemone toxins are listed as mammalian Kv1 channel blockers in the kalium database, which populate all Kv types, except Kv type 5. Each of these types of cnidarian toxins are examined in detail below.

Table 2. Sea anemone peptides directed against Kv1 channel.

Toxin	Source	Inhibited Kv1 Channels	References
Type 1			
ShK	*Stichodactyla helianthus*	Kv1.1, Kv1.3, Kv1.4, 1.6	[106,107]
AeK	*Actinia equina*	^{125}I α-DTX binding to synaptosomal membranes (IC$_{50}$ 22 nM)	[108]
AETX K	*Anemonia erythraea*	^{125}I α-dendrotoxinDTX binding to synaptosomal membranes (IC$_{50}$ 91 nM)	[109]
AsKS	*Anemonia sulcata*	Kv1.2	[110,111]
BcsTX1/2	*Bunodosoma caissarum*	BcsTx1 Kv1.2, Kv1.6 BcsTx2 Kv1.1, Kv1.2, Kv 1.3, Kv1.6, Shaker IR with nM IC$_{50}$	
BgK	*Bunodosoma granulifera*	Kv1.1, Kv1.2, Kv1.3, Kv1.6	[112,113]
HmK	*Heteractis (Radianthus) magnifica*	Kv1.2, Kv1.3	[114,115]
Type 2			
AsKC1	*Anemonia sulcata*	Kv1.2	[111]
AsKC2	*Anemonia sulcata*	Kv1.2	[116]
AsKC3	*Anemonia sulcata*	Kv1.2	[116]
APEXTx1	*Anthopleura elegantissima*	Kv1.1	
SHTXIII	*Stichodactyla haddoni*	^{125}I α-DTXdendrotoxin binding to synaptosomal membranes (IC$_{50}$ 270 nM)	[117]

Table 2. *Cont.*

Toxin	Source	Inhibited Kv1 Channels	References
Type 3			
BDS-I	*Anemonia sulcata*	Kv1.1–5 < 20% inhibition at 10 μM	[116]
APETx1/2/4	*Anthopleura elegantissima*	Kv1.1-6 < 30% inhibition at 100 nM	
PhcrTx2	*Phymanthus crucifer*	Slight inhibition on DRG Kv currents at μM concentrations	[118,119]
Type 4			
SHTX I/II	*Stichodactyla haddoni*	None	
Type 5			
BcsTx3	*Bunodosoma caissarum*	Kv1.1, Kv1.2, Kv 1.3, Kv1.6, Shaker IR	[110]
PhcrTx1	*Phymanthus crucifer*	Slight inhibition on DRG Kv currents at μM concentrations	[120]
Type 6			
AbeTx1	*Actinia bermudensis*	Kv1.1, Kv1.2, Kv1.6, Shaker IR	[121]

3.1. Kv Type 1 Anemone Toxins

Kv type 1 toxins are toxins that include an ShK motif identified from stichodactylatoxin ShK extracted from *Stichodactyla helianthus*. Other VDPs that fall in this family include AeK (*Actinia equina*), AETX K (*Anemonia erythraea*), Kaliseptine AsKS (*Anemonia sulcata*), BcsTXI/II (*Bunodosoma caissarum*), BgK (*Bunodosoma granulifera*), and HmK (*Heteractis magnifica*). They are composed of 34–38 amino acids and cross-linked by three disulfide bridges (3–35, 12–28, and 17–32) [100]; see Figure 4.

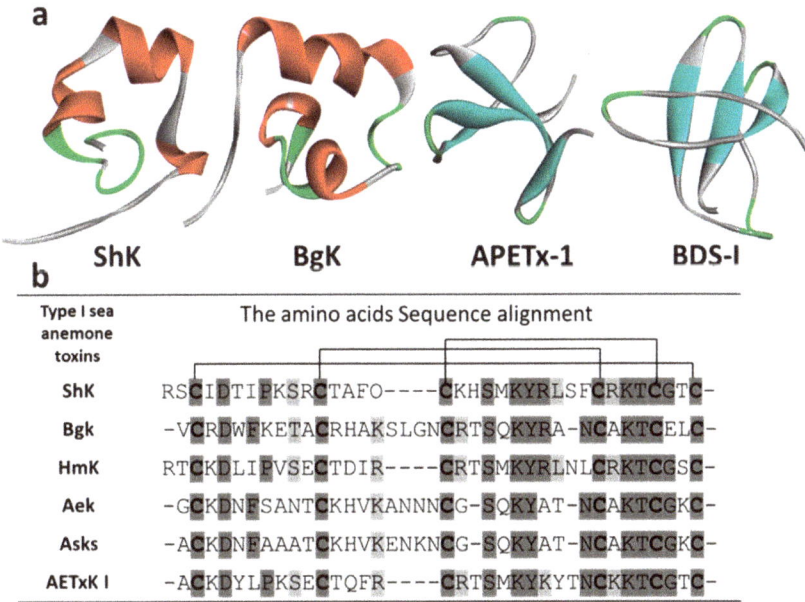

Figure 4. (**a**) Structures of sea anemone peptide toxins ShK (PDB: 1ROO, [53]), BgK (PDB: 1BGK, [46]), APETx-1 (PDB: 1WQK, [122]), and BDS-I (PDB: 2BDS, [123]): The location of the disulfide linkages are shown in green, beta-sheets are in blue, and alpha-helices are in red. (**b**) Sequence alignment of type 1 sea anemone K_V-toxins according to their cysteine framework with the pairings indicated by the lines linking them: Amino acid identity (dark shade) and similarities (light shade) are shown [110].

3.1.1. ShK

One of the first Kv1 channel blockers characterized was ShK (*Stichodactyla helianthus* K$^+$ channel toxin; Figures 2 and 4a [124,125]. ShK potently blocks Kv1.3 and Kv1.1 over Kv1.4 and Kv1.6

channels [106,107]. The amount of ShK found in the *Stichodactyla helianthus* body is relatively small, yet chemical synthesis of the wild-type peptide and its analogs allowed its in-depth study. ShK is a 35-amino-acid peptide with a molecular mass of 4055 Da containing three disulfide-bonded cysteine pairs (C3–C35, C12–C28, and C17–C32) [53,125]. Surface residues of ShK bind at the entrance of the Kv1 channel and block ion conduction by plugging the pore using Lys22 (Figure 2b). The position of the two key binding residues (K22 and Y23) in ShK is conserved in related K^+ channel blocking peptides from other sea anemones (Figure 4b) [46]. Alanine scanning experiments also identified three other amino acids, S20, K22, and Y23, as essential for the binding of ShK to rat brain potassium channels [107]. In T lymphocytes, Kv1.3 channel activity seems to dominate the membrane potential, where high potency block of this current by ShK highlights its potential use as an immunosuppressant [106,107,126]. However, this peptide has strong binding affinity for neuronal Kv1.1 as well as for its bona fide target Kv1.3 in effector-memory T cells [127]. Thus, the identification of ShK analogs that are highly selective for Kv1.3 over Kv1.1 would enable their use in the treatment of autoimmune diseases such as rheumatoid arthritis and diabetes [102]. To address this, much effort has been dedicated to the optimization of ShK's sequence to bias selectivity towards Kv1.3. For example, the N-terminal extension on ShK (EWSS) is 158-fold more selective to Kv1.3 over Kv1.1 [127]. Non-peptide-based modifications of ShK include the addition of a 20 kDa poly(ethylene glycol) in ShK-PEG, which increased ShK selectivity 1000-fold, reaching picomolar potency in whole-blood T cell assays and improved the peptide's half-life in vivo [128].

Albeit with lower potency, ShK also blocks Kv3.2 channel (IC_{50}~0.3 nM, [129]). Hence, the ShK therapeutic scaffold is being exploited for the development of analogs with improved selectivity profiles [130]. More selective analogs for Kv1.1 and Kv1.3 were developed by amino acid replacements with differently charged or non-natural amino acids (ShK-Dap^{22}, IC_{50} 23 pM), analogs containing phospho-tyrosine (ShK-186, IC_{50} 69 pM), and phosphono-phenylalanine (ShK-192, IC_{50} 140 pM), which contain non-protein adducts and hydrolysable phosphorylated residues [115,131]. Such work suggests that selective Kv1.3 antagonists such as ShK-Dap^{22}, for which structural and functional data are available, might represent promising immunosuppressant leads [106,114].

ShK-K-amide is an ShK analog in which an amidated lysine residue has been added to the C-terminus, resulting in potent and selective block of Kv1.3 [132]. ShK inhibits Kv1.3 and Kv1.1 channels with similar potencies (IC_{50} of 9 ± 2 pM and 23 ± 3 pM, respectively). While retaining potency (IC_{50} 26 ± 3 pM) against Kv1.3 channels, ShK-K-amide's affinity for Kv1.1 is greatly reduced (IC_{50} 942 ± 120 pM), thus being 36-fold more selective between these two Kv1 isoforms. It is reasoned that addition of a C-terminal-amidated positive charge by the extra lysine changes the electrostatic interaction between the peptide's C and N-termini, resulting in more favorable interaction with Kv1.3 by allowing arginine 1 to engage with the channel vestibule as well as the previously reported strongly coupled pair R29-S379 in Kv1.3-ShK [127]. However, the extra C-terminal lysine (in ShK-K-amide) disrupts binding with Kv1.1 by apparently altering K18 and R29 interactions with negatively charged residues in the channel.

3.1.2. BgK

BgK is a 37-amino-acid peptide isolated from the sea anemone *Bunodosoma granulifera*, which blocks Kv1.1, Kv1.2, and Kv1.3 channels [112]. BgK is a 37 amino acid peptide crosslinked by three disulfide bridges (C2–C37, C11–C30, and C20–C34), and free C-terminal carboxylate. Both natural and synthetic BgK inhibit binding of ^{125}I-α-DTX to rat brain synaptosomal membranes with nanomolar potency [112]. Corresponding BgK residues (S23, K25, and Y26) are involved in binding to rat brain potassium channels Kv1.1, Kv1.2, Kv1.3, and Kv1.6 [133]. BgK does not select between Kv1.1, Kv1.2, and Kv1.3 channels expressed in *Xenopus* oocytes, displaying quite similar dissociating constants (K_d = 6 nM, 15 nM, and 10 nM, respectively [113]). BgK and ShK share 13 residues and present similar but not exact topologies (Figure 2a) ([46,126] Figure 4b). It has been shown that shortening of K25 side chain by removal of the four methylene groups dramatically decreases the affinity of BgK towards all

Kv1 channels [134]. Mutations at position F6 in BgK reduce potency towards both Kv1.2 and Kv1.3 while not affecting Kv1.1, making BgK-F6A selective for Kv1.1 [135]. BgK-F6A increased miniature excitatory postsynaptic current in neurons while not affecting T-cell activation. This suggests that the Kv1.1 blockade has potential in neuro-inflammatory diseases including multiple sclerosis and stroke and BgK-F6A as a scaffold for drug design.

3.1.3. BcsTx1/2

Two toxins from the venom of *Bunodosoma caissarum* were isolated and named, BcsTX1 and BcsTx2 [110]. These peptides contained the classical three disulfide bonding pattern of Kv type 1 toxins and were screened against a panel of Kv channels, displaying no affinity towards channels outside of the Kv1 subfamily. Both toxins showed differences in their Kv1 selectivity, with BcsTX1 being 10-fold selective for Kv1.2 (~30 nM) over Kv1.6 (~1.6 µM), which in turn was >10-fold selective over other Kv1 channels examined, while BcsTX1 was less selective, displaying the highest affinity for Kv1.6 but less than 10-fold greater than Kv1.1, Kv1.2, and Kv1.3 [110].

3.1.4. Other Kv Type 1 Toxins

Other Kv type 1 sea anemone toxins are known to interact with Kv1 channels; however, little follow has been completed looking at their selectivity or therapeutic potential in depth. The sea anemone *Heteractis magnifica* venom contains the VDP, HmK. It is 35 amino acids long, having an identical molecular weight (MW 4055) to ShK, with 60% homology. HmK is approximately 40% identical to BgK and AsKS (Figure 4b). Partial reduction at acidic pH and rapid alkylation allowed the full assignment of the disulfide linkages (C3–C35, C12–C28, and C17–C32). HmK inhibits the binding of ^{125}I-α-DTX to rat brain synaptosomal membranes with a ~1 nM K_i and block Kv1.2 channels and facilitates neuromuscular junction acetylcholine [114]. Alanine scanning analyses proved that six amino acids (D5, S20, and the dipeptides KY22–23 and KT30–31) are crucial for binding to rat brain Kv channels and perfectly conserved between BgK, ShK AsKS, and HmK [114].

AeK, isolated from *Actinia equine*, is a Kv1 channel toxin that inhibits the binding of ^{125}I-α-DTX rat synaptosomal membranes in a dose-dependent manner with an IC_{50} of 22 nM [108]. The complete amino acid sequence of AeK is composed of 36 amino acid and six cysteine residues. AeK's three disulfides are located between C2–C36, C11–C29, and C20–C33. AeK contains the canonical dyad for Kv channel block formed by K22 and Y23. AeK is similar to AsKS structurally with which it shares 86% sequence homology, 53% with BgK, and 36% with ShK (Figure 4b). However, the selectivity of this peptide has not been addressed functionally.

AsKS, or kaliseptine, is a 36-amino-acid peptide isolated from the sea anemone *Anemonia sulcata* that blocks Kv1 channels and impedes the binding of ^{125}I-α-DTX to receptors in rat brain membrane [111]. AsKS shares 49% sequence homology with BgK toxin ([134] Figure 4b) but differs in two of its cysteine residues (C33 and C36) and the C-terminus. Dendrotoxin I (DTX-I) is a potent blocker of Kv1.1-, Kv1.2-, and Kv1.6-mediated currents in *Xenopus* oocytes. Despite being structurally dissimilar, AsKS appears to share a receptor site in Kv1 channels with the kalicludines (AsKC) and DTX-I. The simple comparison on the capacity of AsKS inhibition for Kv1.2 channel with inhibition ^{125}I-α-dendrotoxin binding to neuronal membranes should be followed with a more in-depth investigation.

The mature AETxK peptide from *Anemonia erythraea* is 34 residues long; six cysteines are paired to form three disulfide bridges (C2–C34, C11–C27, and C16–C31) and presents a canonical Kv channel-blocking dyad comprised of K21 and Y22. AETxK is 59% and 65% homologous to ShK and HmK respectively, whereas it shares 41–44% sequence homology to all other type 1 anemone toxins (Figure 4b). AETxK blocks ^{125}I-α-DTX binding to rat synaptosomal membranes with an estimated IC_{50} of 91 nM [109]. No electrophysiological or related functional data has been reported for this peptide; therefore, its selectivity is unknown [109].

These VDP are all similar to the well-studied ShK; thus, in-depth selectivity profiling is required for these toxins on both homomeric and heteromeric Kv1 channels. These toxins have the potential as scaffolds for therapeutics targeting of autoimmune disorders, stroke, diabetes, multiple sclerosis, and others. None of these toxins have been tested on hetero-tetrameric Kv1 channels and, with their divergent affinities across the Kv1s, may provide interesting routes to discovering selective compounds for various heteromeric Kv1 channels.

3.2. Kv Type 2 Anemone Toxins

Kv type 2 anemone toxins all contain a kunitz-type motif and function as both protease inhibitors and Kv channel blockers. They were first isolated from sea anemones *Anemonia sulcata* and named kalicludines (AsKC1–AsKC3) [130]. However, other Kv type 2 inhibitors have been discovered including APEKTx1 (*Anthopleura elegantissima*) [136] and SHTXIII (*Stichodactyla haddoni*) [117]. When compared to Kv type 1, Kv type 2 anemone toxins typically have lower affinity towards Kv1 channels, making their biological role unclear. They may act to paralyze prey through their dual action protease/Kv channel activity, to provide protection for prey/predator proteases (or, in a similar fashion, to provide protection for their own venom components when injected into their prey/predator), or to act to regulate digestive mechanisms [137]. AsKC1-3 (kalicludines 1–3), are composed of 57–60 amino acid residues with protease inhibitor activity [111]. A mutation at position 19 lowers their inhibitory effect that linked to the sequence homology of BPTI, protein Kunitz-type protease inhibitors [104]. AsKC1 and AsKC2 contain the fully conserved dyad K5/L9 responsible for competing with the DTX-I site in Kv1 channels. They share ~40% amino acid homology with other toxins from venomous animals, such as DTX and BPTI, but AsKC1 and AsKC2 have different specificity from AsKC3 [111,130]. However, further studies should be conducted on the selectivity of these toxins.

In contrast, APEKTx1 has an in-depth study into its selectivity across a variety of ion channels. This study revealed potent activity against Kv1.1 (0.9 nM) with >1000-fold selectivity over other Kv1 channel members, making it an excellent probe into Kv1 channelopathies.

3.3. Kv Type 3 Anemone Toxins

Kv type 3 anemone toxins contain a β-defensin-fold characterized by a short helix or turn followed by a small twisted antiparallel β-sheet. β-defensin are antimicrobial peptides, and anemones have weaponized them as neurotoxins [138] to target not just Kv channels but also Nav and acid sensing ion channels (ASIC) [139,140]. Five Kv type three toxins are shown to have affinity towards Kv1s although very modestly. These include BDS-I (blood depressing substance I from *Anemonia sulcata*), APETx1/2/4 (*Anthopleura elegantissima*), and PhcrTx2 (*Phymanthus crucifer*). BDS-I was first characterized as an antihypertensive and antiviral compound [141]. It was later shown that BDS-I inhibited Kv3.1, Kv3.2, and Kv3.4 with nanomolar concentrations, with only a week inhibitory effect of Kv1.1–5 [116]. BDS-1 has also been shown to inhibit voltage-gated sodium channels in the nanomolar range [142]. Similar to BDS-I, APETx1, 2, and 4 have similar issues with selectivity towards Kv1s. APETx1 and APETx4 are more selective for hERG [118,143], while APETx2 is selective for ASIC channels [138]. PhcrTx2 showed little inhibition of the total DRG Kv channels currents (IC_{50} 6.4 µM) or heterologously expressed Kv1 channels [119]. Currently, no Kv type 3 anemone toxin is specific for Kv1s, suggesting this family of toxins may not be Kv1 therapeutics of potential pharmacological agents. However, future studies will be interesting to address if the Kv type 5 anemone toxins are all antimicrobial and, if so, do they target prokaryotic potassium channels.

3.4. Kv Type 4 Anemone Toxins

Kv type 4 anemone toxins are characterized by a novel fold called boundless β-hairpin. SHTX I (28 residues) and SHTX II (an analog of SHTX I, 28 residues), based on their structure, has been shown that SHTX I and II have only been shown to inhibit binding of ^{125}I-DTX [117] with no channel blocking specificity described. Further studies are required to ascertain selectivity and potency towards Kv1s to assess their future potential as therapeutics or pharmacological tools

3.5. Kv Type 5 Anemone Toxins

Kv type 5 anemone toxins contain the ubiquitous, inhibitor cysteine knot (ICK) motif. BcsTx3 is a 50-amino-acid peptide and Kv toxin extracted from the venom of the sea anemone *Bunodosoma caissarum* with a molecular weight of 5710.52 Da and four disulfide bridges. High identity (65.3% and 63.3%) with BscTx3 and identical positions of cysteine residues have been found in toxins isolated from *Nematostella vectensis* and *Metridium senile*. Another Kv type 5 anemone toxin, PhcrTx1 (*Phymanthus crucifer*), has low affinity modulatory actions on Kv1 channels; however, its main target has been shown to be ASIC channels [120].

Activity investigation of BcsTx3 has been done by Reference [110] on 12 cloned voltage-gated potassium channels and 3 voltage-gated sodium channels. It was shown that BcsTx3 blocks Kv channels Kv1.1, Kv1.2, Kv1.3, Kv1.6, and Shaker IR (inactivation removed) and did not show any activity on sodium channels. The blockage activity of BcsTx3 is not voltage dependent, and the binding site is located at the extracellular side. The lysine and tyrosine functional dyads are absent although present in most of the pore blocker toxins. BcsTx3 binds to Shaker IR through multipoint interaction due to existence of two putative dyads (R5-Y6 and R39-Y40). The evolution of the neurotoxin gene family has been followed by sequencing of the entire genome of *N. vectensis*. It has been shown that peptides in sea anemones responsible for blocking Kv channels evolved at least five times independently but that adaptive evolution took place in a common ancestor [144]. It remains to be seen if any Kv type 5 anemone toxins will provide selectivity within the Kv1 channel family, and thus, any potential as a therapeutic scaffold so far is limited. However, the ICK motif is highly stable, resistant to denaturation and proteolysis [145], which make excellent potential therapeutics if selectivity can be conferred.

3.6. Kv Type 6 Anemone Toxins

Kv type 6 anemone toxins are the shortest of Kv-type sea anemone toxins and contain a proline-hinged asymmetric β-hairpin fold. AbeTx1 is a toxin with a unique primary structure isolated from nematocysts of the sea anemone *Actinia bermudensis*. It is short flexible random-coil-like conformational peptide chain of 17 amino acids with a tendency to form β-sheet (aromatic or aliphatic amino acids are not present, but it contains a high proportion of Lys and Arg, and two disulfide bridges between C1–C4 and C2–C3) [121].

The activity of AbeTx1 was tested on 12 subtypes of Kv channels (Kv1.1–Kv1.6; Kv2.1; Kv3.1; Kv4.2; Kv4.3; Kv11.1; and Shaker IR) and three voltage-gated sodium channels (Na$_V$1.2, Na$_V$1.4, and BgNa$_V$). It has been shown that AbeTx1 is selective for Shaker-related K$^+$ channels and is capable of inhibiting K$^+$ currents by blocking the K$^+$ current of Kv1.2 or by altering activation of Kv1.1 and Kv1.6 channels. AbeTx1 showed no activity on sodium channels, but the same concentration (3 μM) inhibits the current of Kv1.1, Kv1.2, Kv1.3, Kv1.6, and Shaker IR channels [121]. It is known that the mechanism of Kv channel toxins is multipoint interaction binding to ring based amino acid, and due to the presence of six such amino acid rings (R1, R9, R11, K3, K7, and K13), AbeTx1 toxins interact with Kv1.1 and Kv1.6 channels. Electrophysiological experiments were performed to determine the mechanism of action, and it has been discovered that probably AbeTx1 toxin binds on the outer side of Kv1.2 and Kv1.6 channels since its effect is reversible (current was recovered). Competitive binding experiments with TEA showed that binding sites for both ligands are not overlapping completely on Kv1.1, which is not the case with Kv1.6 channels due to less voltage dependence of blockage of Kv1.1 with membrane depolarization [121].

Also, alanine point-mutated analogs were tested on Kv1.1 and Kv1.6 channels. Six synthetic analogs were used to test a multipoint interaction of the toxin to the channel's binding site, and it has been shown that loss of the side chains will lead to decreasing activity of analogs [121].

4. Non-Peptidyl Kv1 Channel Inhibitors

4.1. Gambierol

One of the non-peptidyl toxins from the ciguatera group (CigTXs) is gambierol (Figure 5), marine polycyclic ether toxin isolated from marine dinoflagellate *Gambierdiscus toxicus* showing acute toxicity in mice (LD_{50} = 50 mg/Kg, ip; [146]). These CigTXs are accumulated throughout the marine food chain, causing hypotension, bradycardia, respiratory difficulties, and paralysis [147]. Although CigTXs are toxic for Nav channels, gambierol inhibits only Kv1 potassium channels [147,148].

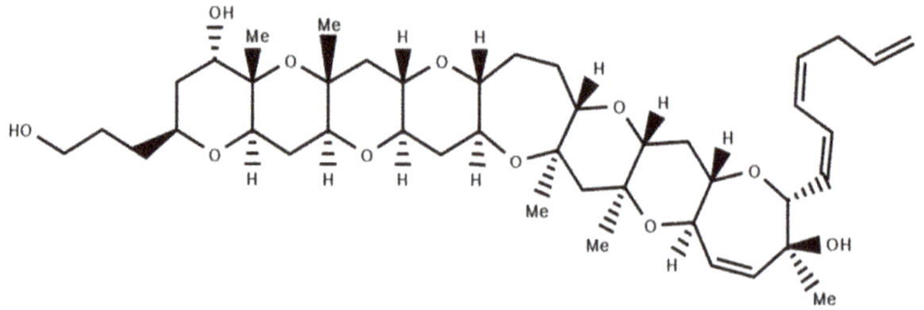

Figure 5. Structure of Gambierol toxin showing the eight polyether rings [129]: Me indicates a methyl group.

Gambierol is lipophilic and can pass through the cell membrane. This was confirmed as Gambierol inhibited closed channels no matter which side the toxin was applied [148]. Gambierol has heptacyclic and tetracyclic analogs that are specific inhibitors for the Kv1.2 channel expressed in CHO cells with IC_{50}s of 0.75, 7.6, and 28 nM, respectively [146]. However, the dose-dependent leak current induced by these compounds might be behind their cytotoxic effect. Screening of Gambierol against other Kv channels revealed that Kv2 and Kv4 were insensitive to 1 μM gambierol but fully repressed Kv3.1 channels [149]. The same study showed ~70% inhibition of K^+-mediated currents by Kv1.4 using 100 nM Gambierol.

According to Kopljar, et al., 2009 [149], Kv3 channels inhibition occurs when channels are deactivated, suggesting a mechanism related to gating modification. Swapping of the S5–S6 linker between Kv3.1 and Kv2.1 channels gave no differences in selectivity of gambierol to either of the channels, indicating that gambierol is not an external pore blocker. Kv1 and Kv3 channels contain threonine residues in the inner permeation pathway, while the insensitive Kv2 and Kv4 channels have valine at the same position. After the replacement of threonine with different moieties, it was confirmed that hydrogen bonding capable amino acids (serine and lysine) contribute to the high affinity of gambierol to Kv3.1 channels. The T427 residue between the S5 and S6 segments of Kv3.1 channels interacts with one of the ether oxygens of the toxin, thereby inhibiting permeation of K^+ ions and stabilizing the closed state.

4.2. Aplysiatoxin Derivatives

Marine cyanobacteria are a source of many toxins, including a recently discovered group of Kv1.5 blockers called Aplysiatoxins (ATXs). ATXs and related analogs, namely Oscillatoxins and nhatrangins (Figure 6), are 27 bioactive dermatoxins polyketide compounds that were isolated from several marine cyanobacteria species with antiproliferative activity, tumor-promoting properties, proinflammatory actions, and antiviral activity (see Reference [150]). According to the structural characteristics, ATXs were divided into three categories: (1) the ABC tricyclic ring systems with carbon numbers of 6/12/6, 6/10/6, and 6/6/6 (e.g., Debromoaplysiatoxins and neo-debromoaplysiatoxins) [151]; (2) the AB spirobicyclic ring system (e.g., Oscillatoxin D) [152], and (3) acyclic structures such as Nhatrangins [153].

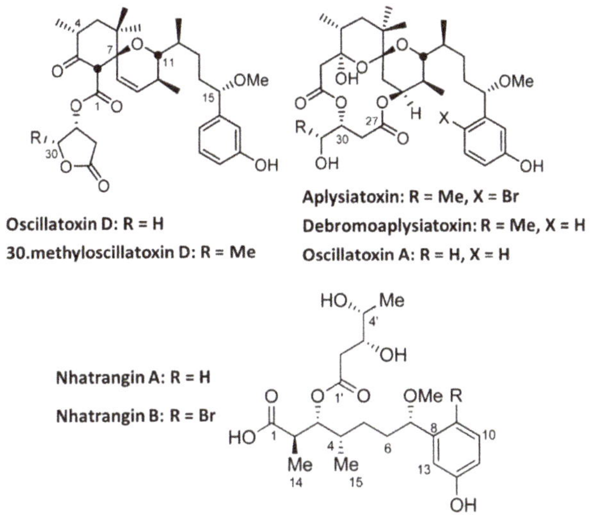

Figure 6. Structure of representative Aplysiatoxin derivatives from References [152,153]: Me indicates a methyl group.

In addition to their various structures, ATX derivatives exhibit selectivity and potency against Kv1.5 channels, a possible pivotal target for new treatment of atrial tachyarrhymias with minimal potential for deleterious side effect [151,154,155]. Although further studies are still ongoing to establish the Kv1.5 inhibition mechanism by these various bioactive compounds, researchers suggested two mechanisms. One is the direct ion channel modulation by direct blocking of the pore. The other proposed mechanism is the indirect modulation of the Kv channel by activating protein kinase C [154].

5. Kv1-Active Toxins in Research and Drug Discovery

Venom-derived toxins have been paramount in the identification and study of ion channels. Neuronal Kv1 heteromeric complexes were first recognized thanks to snake dendrotoxins and were identified by isoform-specific antibody fractionation [36,37,40]. We have learned that the majority of Kv1 channel complexes present in the nervous system are hetero-tetrameric combinations of Kv1 α-subunits, while only a small fraction of channels are homo-tetramers (e.g., neuronal: Kv1.2 and 1.4; immune system Kv1.3). The composition, stoichiometries, and subunit arrangements of Kv1 complexes expressed in different tissues and cells remains to be fully identified. As seen in the sections above, many of the venom-derived toxins published have not been screened against homomeric Kv1 channels and thus lack information of biological potential. To understand the therapeutic potential of these toxins, it is necessary to study their effects on relevant heteromeric Kv channel complexes. This requires efforts that include but are not limited to the generation and functional characterization of concatenated (or tandem) hetero-tetramers [156,157], as proxies of the physiological targets, in bioactive-driven molecular tool development and drug discovery.

By examining venom-derived peptides on hetero-tetrameric Kv1, it has recently been discovered that some VDP display significantly higher potencies for heteromeric Kv1s than those with the same contributing homomeric channel isoforms. For example, testing of conotoxin κM-RIIIJ over 12 different heterodimers containing Kv1.2 subunits, Cordeiro et al. showed that RIIIJ was most potent against Kv1.1/Kv1.2 heterodimers without apparent regard for their arrangement, showing significant discrimination against other heterodimeric constructs including those formed by association of Kv1.2 with Kv1.5 or Kv1.6. Further functional analyses showed that RIIIJ was indeed ~100 more potent against hetero-tetramers made of three copies of Kv1.2 α-subunits and one of either Kv1.1 or Kv1.6 in a

3:1 stoichiometry [82]. This detailed functional and biochemical characterization then enabled the use of RIIIJ as a molecular tool for the classification of live large DRG neurons into six discrete functional populations [83]. An approach that can be exploited to accelerate the classification and study of other cell types within mixed population.

The thorough functional characterization of Conkunitzin-S1 allowed the identification of Kv1.7 channels in pancreatic beta cells as contributors in glucose-stimulated insulin secretion [12]. As shown for the RIIIJ/Kv1.2 interactions, the presence of the Kv1.7 α-subunit confers sensitivity to Conk-S1 to a Kv1 hetero-tetramer. In contrast to RIIIJ, Conk-S1 (and Conk-S2) appears to be able to discriminate different Kv1 targets based on their relative positioning [12]. Thus, hinting to the Conks' potential as molecular tools in the study of heteromeric Kv1 channels in native tissues.

The thorough characterization and in vivo study of Conk-S1 was possible due to the production of high yields by recombinant expression of the peptide in *E. coli* [52], which guarantees inexpensive production. Much like monomeric insulin, Conk-S1 is a small peptide (<10 kDa) in which therapeutic potential for the treatment of hyperglycemic disorders is supported principally by its effectiveness, in vivo and ex vivo, to enhance insulin secretion and lower glucose levels in a strictly glucose dependent manner because the targeted Kv1.7 channel opens at depolarized potentials that are achieved upon increases in blood glucose (i.e., postprandial). Consequently, Conk-S1 treatment appears to modulate pancreatic β-beta cell excitability only at stimulatory glucose concentrations where bursting electrical activity is observed but not at low/basal glucose concentrations, eliminating the risk of hypoglycemia [12]. This is advantageous because the current drugs used to ameliorate diabetes are effective at lowering blood glucose but do so regardless of the basal conditions. Hence, acute, delayed, and persistent hypoglycemia constitutes the most frequent adverse effect associated with sulfonylureas (K_{ATP} channel inhibitors) and insulin-based therapies, obliging frequent monitoring of blood glucose concentrations [158]. Furthermore, intraperitoneal Conk-S1 injections neither affected basal glucose levels nor produced adverse cardiovascular or neurological side effects in vivo [12], highlighting the safety of targeting Kv1.7 channels. Nevertheless, the identification and validation of biological target(s) as well as prediction of biological activities of Conk-S1 must be verified in alternative systems including animal models in order to ascertain the mechanism of action behind Conk-S1's pro-insulinogenic effects. Further, Structure-Activity Relationship (SAR)-aided computational work would be useful to aid functional refinements in the selectivity and potency of Conk-S1 for its development as a therapeutic to minimize potential side effects and to decrease production costs.

Much has been done in the case of the anemone toxins. For instance, ShK is considered the most potent blocker for Kv1.3 channels with an IC_{50} of 10 pM [106]. However, it also potently blocks Kv1.1, 1.4, and 1.6 channels [131,159]. Kv1.3 has been shown to be a potential target of immune-modulators; hence, in order to enhance its selectivity over other targeted Kv1 isoforms, analogs of ShK have been generated [115]. These efforts paved the way for the development of a leading blocker called ShK-186, which has a 100-fold improvement in selectivity for Kv1.3 over Kv1.1, 1.4, and 1.6 channels [160]. Currently known as dalazatide, it successfully passed phase 1 clinical trials in 2016 and entered phase 2 in 2018 for the treatment of several autoimmune diseases like inclusion body myositis, lupus, multiple sclerosis, psoriasis, rheumatoid arthritis, type 1 diabetes, and inflammatory bowel diseases. Promising newer generation, ShK analogues are currently under development [102].

6. Challenges and Outlook

In this review, a conscious attempt was made to provide an overview of those Kv1-targeted marine bioactives for which functional data including potency and selectivity has been reported. The availability of such information has allowed their development as molecular tools, as are the cases of κ-RIIIJ and Conk-S1, and therapeutically promising pharmacological scaffolds like ShK or Conk-S1. The wealth of marine bioactive molecules targeting Kv1 channels is immense, yet the vast majority has been characterized only at the sequence level. The collection of marine toxins presented here was focused around Kv1 channel modulatory activity. However, the selectivity profiles of most marine toxins, both the peptides and non-peptides, are absent or inadequate; hence, further work is necessary to assess their real potential as research tools and therapeutics.

Competition binding data is customarily reported for venom-derived compounds, but this is at best indicative of their potential bioactivity. Comprehensive functional profiling is fundamental to attest to the potential of the abundance of toxins identified, albeit it is not achieved without substantial challenges. First, the primary sequence of venom derived peptides is used to predict their 3D structure and to guide inference of potential targets. Unfortunately, similar scaffolds are often used to target across families of ion channels and enzymes; therefore, functional verification is an absolute requirement. Second, most selectivity screens to determine specificity of Kv1-targeted compounds are limited to their functional assessment in homo-tetrameric Kv1 channels assembled upon expression of a single α-subunit in heterologous systems. Most native Kv channels are not homomeric but heteromeric complexes formed by up to four different α-subunits, as is the case of the CNS and PNS Kv channels, and thus, natural bioactive species such as marine toxins and VDPs have evolved to target heteromeric combinations. These natural molecules have been selected through evolution to serve as molecular tools for the study of native Kv channels. Furthermore, the study of the molecular determinants guiding marine bioactive targeting of heteromeric Kv channels would aid the design of pharmacological agents for the treatment of various channelopathies.

κ-conotoxins, such as RIIIK, RIIIJ, Conk-S1, and Conk-S2 toxins, have been shown to discriminate among targets based on heteromeric composition and order of connectivity [12]. Naturally evolved K+ channel-targeted ligands may become instrumental in the study of heteromeric Kv1 channels in live biological systems allowing facile determination of composition and physiological function. Efforts must be made towards bioactivity determination in hetero-multimeric Kv1 channels in heterologous systems and by coupling functional studies with single cell transcriptomics/proteomics of primary cultures. The findings from such work would provide invaluable to the development of leading drugs against heteromeric channels associated with Kv1 channelopathies [25].

VDP inhibitors select among heteromeric Kv1 channel targets according to their α-subunit identities, their stoichiometry, and their arrangement by binding across monomeric boundaries. This could account for the diversity of selectivity "fingerprints" observed in native cells/tissues and highlights marine toxin relevance as molecular tools and pharmacological applications. The potency and selectivity of bioactives found in nature provides a wealth of scaffolds with therapeutic potential. From one side, the molecular understanding of the ion channel pore structure was revealed by using natural peptide-based toxins as molecular probes. On the other hand, better understanding of the Kv1 channels as drug targets for the treatment of disease is crucial for developing promising therapies.

Comparatively speaking, few marine toxins have been functionally explored in enough depth to be considered for research or clinical purposes. Only a few labs in the world have full capabilities to perform all: discovery, synthesis/production, functional characterization, and experimentation in animal models. Therefore, collaboration between expert labs from each and all disciplines involved is an absolute requirement for the advance of the field.

Despite the high interest in the discovery of novel marine toxins, many challenges exist in advancing them into therapeutically active compounds. Amongst those challenges, the development of adequate transferable human assays to assess compound's selectivity and off-target activity is paramount. Selectivity and SAR screens are time and labor intensive, requiring large amounts of pure material. For example, synthesis and purification of biologically active peptides are ridden with numerous potential pitfalls such as the selection of the optimal prokaryotic or eukaryotic expression host (bacteria, yeast, or mammalian cell lines). The production of recombinant proteins has predominantly used bacterial expression due the ability to generate high protein yields from large volume cultures of fast-growing, low-cost bacteria [161,162]. However, when the protein products involve eukaryotic posttranslational modifications, mammalian or insect cells become the system of choice. Often, functionally, many marine peptides require proper folding supported by their cysteine connectivity, which can curtail yields of active proteins [163] and/or incorporate posttranslational modifications critical for their activity. Despite the advantages of eukaryotic expression systems, higher production costs preclude their use [164]. Recently, periplasmic peptide expression in *E. coli* has made use of the oxidizing environment to produce folded peptides (i.e., Reference [165]). While this has the potential to speed up protein production, it is limited as targeting across the cytoplasmic membrane can substantially limit periplasmic yields [166,167]. Marine non-peptidyl compounds also pose challenges inherent to their chemistry and organisms that produce them [168]. However, once production of marine compounds is achieved, their stability, formulation, delivery, and antigenicity need to be overcome. Despite these limitations, the potential therapeutic abilities of marine natural products are unquestionable. Successful examples include Zinconotide (Prialt, sever chronic pain), Cytarabine (Cytosar-U, chemotherapy medication), Vidarabine (Vira-A, antiviral drug), Brentuximab Vedotin (Adcetris, chemotherapy medication), Eribulin Mesylate (Halaven, chemotherapy medication), Omega-3-acid ethyl esters (Lovaza, diet and exercise drug which reduces triglycerides), Trabectedin (Yondelis, chemotherapy medication), Fludarabine Phosphate (Fludara, chemotherapy medication), Nelarabine (Arranon, chemotherapy medication), and Iota-carrageenan (carragelose, Antiviral drug), with ~30 in various clinical phase I-IV trials (for a recent review, see Reference [169]).

Marine toxins remain a relatively under-explored source of bioactives targeting Kv1 channels. Technological advances in transcriptomics and proteogenomic will enable the expedited identification of novel marine toxin repertoires, will explore the diversity of their function based on known peptide scaffold, and will understand the relationships of structure-function aspects of these toxins with much more still that remains to be discovered. Importantly, bioactive function can only be determined experimentally. The use of marine toxins and novel, integrative strategies provide powerful approaches to functionally define specific cellular types underlying physiology in health and diseased states. Given the laborious nature of electrophysiological recordings, high-throughput functional assessment platforms involving automated patch clamp are fundamental for substantial output increase in the discovery of novel ion-channel targeting molecules and the advancement of the venom-derived drug discovery field.

Author Contributions: Conceptualization, A.A.-S. and R.K.F.-U.; software and analysis, G.K.K.; visualization and figures design, G.K.K.; R.K.F.-U. and A.A.-S. All the authors contributed to the writing, editing and drafting the manuscript; All authors have read and agreed to the published version of the manuscript.

Funding: This review received no external funding.

Acknowledgments: A special thanks to Teresa Carlomagno (Leibniz Universität Hannover) and Stefan Becker (Max Planck Institute for Biophysical Chemistry, Göttingen) for providing the PDB structure file for κM-RIIIK.

Conflicts of Interest: The authors declare no conflict of interest.

References

1. Hille, B. *Ion channels of excitable membranes*, 3rd ed.; Sunderland, Mass. Sinauer: New York, NY, USA, 2001.
2. Gutman, G.A.; Chandy, K.G.; Grissmer, S.; Lazdunski, M.; McKinnon, D.; Pardo, L.A.; Robertson, G.A.; Rudy, B.; Sanguinetti, M.C.; Stuhmer, W.; et al. International Union of Pharmacology. LIII. Nomenclature and molecular relationships of voltage-gated potassium channels. *Pharmacol. Rev.* **2005**, *57*, 473–508. [CrossRef] [PubMed]
3. Rudy, B. Diversity and ubiquity of K channels. *Neuroscience* **1988**, *25*, 729–749. [CrossRef]
4. Vacher, H.; Mohapatra, D.P.; Trimmer, J.S. Localization and targeting of voltage-dependent ion channels in mammalian central neurons. *Physiol. Rev.* **2008**, *88*, 1407–1447. [CrossRef] [PubMed]
5. Barry, D.M.; Trimmer, J.S.; Merlie, J.P.; Nerbonne, J.M. Differential expression of voltage-gated K^+ channel subunits in adult rat heart. Relation to functional K^+ channels? *Circ. Res.* **1995**, *77*, 361–369. [CrossRef] [PubMed]
6. Kalman, K.; Nguyen, A.; Tseng-Crank, J.; Dukes, I.D.; Chandy, G.; Hustad, C.M.; Copeland, N.G.; Jenkins, N.A.; Mohrenweiser, H.; Brandriff, B.; et al. Genomic organization, chromosomal localization, tissue distribution, and biophysical characterization of a novel mammalian Shaker-related voltage-gated potassium channel, Kv1.7. *J. Biol. Chem.* **1998**, *273*, 5851–5857. [CrossRef] [PubMed]

7.   Matsubara, H.; Liman, E.R.; Hess, P.; Koren, G. Pretranslational mechanisms determine the type of potassium channels expressed in the rat skeletal and cardiac muscles. *J. Biol. Chem.* **1991**, *266*, 13324–13328.

8.   Bose, T.; Cieslar-Pobuda, A.; Wiechec, E. Role of ion channels in regulating Ca^{2+} homeostasis during the interplay between immune and cancer cells. *Cell Death Dis.* **2015**, *6*, e1648. [CrossRef]

9.   Dubois, J.M.; Rouzaire-Dubois, B. The influence of cell volume changes on tumour cell proliferation. *Eur. Biophys. J.* **2004**, *33*, 227–232. [CrossRef]

10.   Rouzaire-Dubois, B.; Dubois, J.M. A quantitative analysis of the role of K^+ channels in mitogenesis of neuroblastoma cells. *Cell. Signal.* **1991**, *3*, 333–339. [CrossRef]

11.   Koo, G.C.; Blake, J.T.; Talento, A.; Nguyen, M.; Lin, S.; Sirotina, A.; Shah, K.; Mulvany, K.; Hora, D., Jr.; Cunningham, P.; et al. Blockade of the voltage-gated potassium channel Kv1.3 inhibits immune responses in vivo. *J. Immunol.* **1997**, *158*, 5120–5128.

12.   Finol-Urdaneta, R.K.; Remedi, M.S.; Raasch, W.; Becker, S.; Clark, R.B.; Struver, N.; Pavlov, E.; Nichols, C.G.; French, R.J.; Terlau, H. Block of Kv1.7 potassium currents increases glucose-stimulated insulin secretion. *EMBO Mol. Med.* **2012**, *4*, 424–434. [CrossRef] [PubMed]

13.   Long, S.B.; Campbell, E.B.; Mackinnon, R. Crystal structure of a mammalian voltage-dependent Shaker family K^+ channel. *Science* **2005**, *309*, 897–903. [CrossRef] [PubMed]

14.   Kurata, H.T.; Fedida, D. A structural interpretation of voltage-gated potassium channel inactivation. *Prog. Biophys. Mol. Biol.* **2006**, *92*, 185–208. [CrossRef] [PubMed]

15.   Bahring, R.; Covarrubias, M. Mechanisms of closed-state inactivation in voltage-gated ion channels. *J. Physiol.* **2011**, *589 (Pt 3)*, 461–479. [CrossRef]

16.   Aldrich, R.W. Fifty years of inactivation. *Nature* **2001**, *411*, 643–644. [CrossRef] [PubMed]

17.   Fan, C.; Sukomon, N.; Flood, E.; Allen, T.W.; Nimigean, C.M. Ball-and-chain inactivation in a calcium-gated potassium channel. *Nature* **2020**.

18.   Pau, V.; Zhou, Y.; Ramu, Y.; Xu, Y.; Lu, Z. Crystal structure of an inactivated mutant mammalian voltage-gated K^+ channel. *Nat. Struct. Mol. Biol.* **2017**, *24*, 857–865. [CrossRef]

19.   Hoshi, T.; Armstrong, C.M. C-type inactivation of voltage-gated K^+ channels: Pore constriction or dilation? *J. Gen. Physiol.* **2013**, *141*, 151–160. [CrossRef]

20.   Valiyaveetil, F.I. A glimpse into the C-type-inactivated state for a Potassium Channel. *Nat. Struct. Mol. Biol.* **2017**, *24*, 787–788. [CrossRef]

21.   Sahoo, N.; Hoshi, T.; Heinemann, S.H. Oxidative modulation of voltage-gated potassium channels. *Antioxid. Redox Signal.* **2014**, *21*, 933–952. [CrossRef]

22.   Finol-Urdaneta, R.K.; Struver, N.; Terlau, H. Molecular and Functional Differences between Heart mKv1.7 Channel Isoforms. *J. Gen. Physiol.* **2006**, *128*, 133–145. [CrossRef]

23.   Al-Sabi, A.; Kaza, S.K.; Dolly, J.O.; Wang, J. Pharmacological characteristics of Kv1.1- and Kv1.2-containing channels are influenced by the stoichiometry and positioning of their alpha subunits. *Biochem. J.* **2013**, *454*, 101–108. [CrossRef] [PubMed]

24.   Kavanaugh, M.P.; Hurst, R.S.; Yakel, J.; Varnum, M.D.; Adelman, J.P.; North, R.A. Multiple subunits of a voltage-dependent potassium channel contribute to the binding site for tetraethylammonium. *Neuron* **1992**, *8*, 493–497. [CrossRef]

25.   Wulff, H.; Castle, N.A.; Pardo, L.A. Voltage-gated potassium channels as therapeutic targets. *Nat. Rev. Drug Discov.* **2009**, *8*, 982–1001. [CrossRef] [PubMed]

26.   Alexander, S.P.H.; Kelly, E.; Mathie, A.; Peters, J.A.; Veale, E.L.; Armstrong, J.F.; Faccenda, E.; Harding, S.D.; Pawson, A.J.; Sharman, J.L.; et al. The Concise Guide To Pharmacology 2019/20: Introduction and Other Protein Targets. *Br. J. Pharmacol.* **2019**, *176* (Suppl. 1), S1–S20. [CrossRef]

27.   Ovsepian, S.V.; LeBerre, M.; Steuber, V.; O'Leary, V.B.; Leibold, C.; Oliver Dolly, J. Distinctive role of KV1.1 subunit in the biology and functions of low threshold K^+ channels with implications for neurological disease. *Pharmacol. Ther.* **2016**, *159*, 93–101. [CrossRef]

28.   Parcej, D.N.; Scott, V.E.; Dolly, J.O. Oligomeric properties of alpha-dendrotoxin-sensitive potassium ion channels purified from bovine brain. *Biochemistry* **1992**, *31*, 11084–11088. [CrossRef]

29.   Pongs, O.; Schwarz, J.R. Ancillary subunits associated with voltage-dependent K^+ channels. *Physiol. Rev.* **2010**, *90*, 755–796. [CrossRef]

30.   Coetzee, W.A.; Amarillo, Y.; Chiu, J.; Chow, A.; Lau, D.; McCormack, T.; Moreno, H.; Nadal, M.S.; Ozaita, A.; Pountney, D.; et al. Molecular diversity of K^+ channels. *Ann. N. Y. Acad. Sci.* **1999**, *868*, 233–285. [CrossRef]

31. Panyi, G.; Deutsch, C. Assembly and suppression of endogenous Kv1.3 channels in human T cells. *J. Gen. Physiol.* **1996**, *107*, 409–420. [CrossRef]
32. Shen, N.V.; Pfaffinger, P.J. Molecular recognition and assembly sequences involved in the subfamily-specific assembly of voltage-gated K$^+$ channel subunit proteins. *Neuron* **1995**, *14*, 625–633. [CrossRef]
33. Xu, J.; Yu, W.; Jan, Y.N.; Jan, L.Y.; Li, M. Assembly of voltage-gated potassium channels. Conserved hydrophilic motifs determine subfamily-specific interactions between the alpha-subunits. *J. Biol. Chem.* **1995**, *270*, 24761–24768. [CrossRef] [PubMed]
34. Tu, L.; Deutsch, C. Evidence for dimerization of dimers in K$^+$ channel assembly. *Biophys. J.* **1999**, *76*, 2004–2017. [CrossRef]
35. Stuhmer, W.; Ruppersberg, J.P.; Schroter, K.H.; Sakmann, B.; Stocker, M.; Giese, K.P.; Perschke, A.; Baumann, A.; Pongs, O. Molecular basis of functional diversity of voltage-gated potassium channels in mammalian brain. *EMBO J.* **1989**, *8*, 3235–3244. [CrossRef] [PubMed]
36. Coleman, S.K.; Newcombe, J.; Pryke, J.; Dolly, J.O. Subunit composition of Kv1 channels in human CNS. *J. Neurochem.* **1999**, *73*, 849–858. [CrossRef]
37. Koch, R.O.; Wanner, S.G.; Koschak, A.; Hanner, M.; Schwarzer, C.; Kaczorowski, G.J.; Slaughter, R.S.; Garcia, M.L.; Knaus, H.G. Complex subunit assembly of neuronal voltage-gated K$^+$ channels. Basis for high-affinity toxin interactions and pharmacology. *J. Biol. Chem.* **1997**, *272*, 27577–27581. [CrossRef]
38. Koschak, A.; Bugianesi, R.M.; Mitterdorfer, J.; Kaczorowski, G.J.; Garcia, M.L.; Knaus, H.G. Subunit composition of brain voltage-gated potassium channels determined by hongotoxin-1, a novel peptide derived from Centruroides limbatus venom. *J. Biol. Chem.* **1998**, *273*, 2639–2644. [CrossRef]
39. Ruppersberg, J.P.; Schroter, K.H.; Sakmann, B.; Stocker, M.; Sewing, S.; Pongs, O. Heteromultimeric channels formed by rat brain potassium-channel proteins. *Nature* **1990**, *345*, 535–537. [CrossRef]
40. Shamotienko, O.G.; Parcej, D.N.; Dolly, J.O. Subunit combinations defined for K$^+$ channel Kv1 subtypes in synaptic membranes from bovine brain. *Biochemistry* **1997**, *36*, 8195–8201. [CrossRef]
41. Schendel, V.; Rash, L.D.; Jenner, R.A.; Undheim, E.A.B. The Diversity of Venom: The Importance of Behavior and Venom System Morphology in Understanding Its Ecology and Evolution. *Toxins (Basel)* **2019**, *11*, 666. [CrossRef]
42. Mouhat, S.; Andreotti, N.; Jouirou, B.; Sabatier, J.M. Animal toxins acting on voltage-gated potassium channels. *Curr. Pharm. Des.* **2008**, *14*, 2503–2518. [CrossRef]
43. Eriksson, M.A.; Roux, B. Modeling the structure of agitoxin in complex with the Shaker K$^+$ channel: A computational approach based on experimental distance restraints extracted from thermodynamic mutant cycles. *Biophys. J.* **2002**, *83*, 2595–2609. [CrossRef]
44. Gao, Y.D.; Garcia, M.L. Interaction of agitoxin 2, charybdotoxin, and iberiotoxin with potassium channels: Selectivity between voltage-gated and Maxi-K channels. *Proteins* **2003**, *52*, 146–154. [CrossRef] [PubMed]
45. Miller, C. The charybdotoxin family of K$^+$ channel-blocking peptides. *Neuron* **1995**, *15*, 5–10. [CrossRef]
46. Dauplais, M.; Lecoq, A.; Song, J.; Cotton, J.; Jamin, N.; Gilquin, B.; Roumestand, C.; Vita, C.; de Medeiros, C.L.; Rowan, E.G.; et al. On the convergent evolution of animal toxins. Conservation of a diad of functional residues in potassium channel-blocking toxins with unrelated structures. *J. Biol. Chem.* **1997**, *272*, 4302–4309. [CrossRef]
47. Gilquin, B.; Racape, J.; Wrisch, A.; Visan, V.; Lecoq, A.; Grissmer, S.; Menez, A.; Gasparini, S. Structure of the BgK-Kv1.1 complex based on distance restraints identified by double mutant cycles. Molecular basis for convergent evolution of Kv1 channel blockers. *J. Biol. Chem.* **2002**, *277*, 37406–37413. [CrossRef]
48. Savarin, P.; Guenneugues, M.; Gilquin, B.; Lamthanh, H.; Gasparini, S.; Zinn-Justin, S.; Menez, A. Three-dimensional structure of kappa-conotoxin PVIIA, a novel potassium channel-blocking toxin from cone snails. *Biochemistry* **1998**, *37*, 5407–5416. [CrossRef]
49. Srinivasan, K.N.; Sivaraja, V.; Huys, I.; Sasaki, T.; Cheng, B.; Kumar, T.K.; Sato, K.; Tytgat, J.; Yu, C.; San, B.C.; et al. kappa-Hefutoxin1, a novel toxin from the scorpion Heterometrus fulvipes with unique structure and function. Importance of the functional diad in potassium channel selectivity. *J. Biol. Chem.* **2002**, *277*, 30040–30047. [CrossRef]
50. Jouirou, B.; Mouhat, S.; Andreotti, N.; De Waard, M.; Sabatier, J.M. Toxin determinants required for interaction with voltage-gated K$^+$ channels. *Toxicon* **2004**, *43*, 909–914. [CrossRef]

51. Al-Sabi, A.; Lennartz, D.; Ferber, M.; Gulyas, J.; Rivier, J.E.; Olivera, B.M.; Carlomagno, T.; Terlau, H. KappaM-conotoxin RIIIK, structural and functional novelty in a K$^+$ channel antagonist. *Biochemistry* **2004**, *43*, 8625–8635. [CrossRef]

52. Bayrhuber, M.; Vijayan, V.; Ferber, M.; Graf, R.; Korukottu, J.; Imperial, J.; Garrett, J.E.; Olivera, B.M.; Terlau, H.; Zweckstetter, M.; et al. Conkunitzin-S1 is the first member of a new Kunitz-type neurotoxin family. Structural and functional characterization. *J. Biol. Chem.* **2005**, *280*, 23766–23770. [CrossRef]

53. Tudor, J.E.; Pallaghy, P.K.; Pennington, M.W.; Norton, R.S. Solution structure of ShK toxin, a novel potassium channel inhibitor from a sea anemone. *Nat. Struct. Biol.* **1996**, *3*, 317–320. [CrossRef]

54. Takahashi, H.; Kim, J.I.; Min, H.J.; Sato, K.; Swartz, K.J.; Shimada, I. Solution structure of hanatoxin1, a gating modifier of voltage-dependent K$^+$ channels: Common surface features of gating modifier toxins. *J. Mol. Biol.* **2000**, *297*, 771–780. [CrossRef] [PubMed]

55. de Vries, S.J.; van Dijk, M.; Bonvin, A.M. The HADDOCK web server for data-driven biomolecular docking. *Nat. Protoc.* **2010**, *5*, 883–897. [CrossRef] [PubMed]

56. van Zundert, G.C.P.; Rodrigues, J.; Trellet, M.; Schmitz, C.; Kastritis, P.L.; Karaca, E.; Melquiond, A.S.J.; van Dijk, M.; de Vries, S.J.; Bonvin, A. The HADDOCK2.2 Web Server: User-Friendly Integrative Modeling of Biomolecular Complexes. *J. Mol. Biol.* **2016**, *428*, 720–725. [CrossRef] [PubMed]

57. DeLano Scientific. *The PyMOL Molecular Graphics System*; DeLano Scientific: Palo Alto, CA, USA, 2002.

58. Kalia, J.; Milescu, M.; Salvatierra, J.; Wagner, J.; Klint, J.K.; King, G.F.; Olivera, B.M.; Bosmans, F. From foe to friend: Using animal toxins to investigate ion channel function. *J. Mol. Biol.* **2015**, *427*, 158–175. [CrossRef]

59. Swartz, K.J.; MacKinnon, R. Hanatoxin modifies the gating of a voltage-dependent K$^+$ channel through multiple binding sites. *Neuron* **1997**, *18*, 665–673. [CrossRef]

60. Karbat, I.; Altman-Gueta, H.; Fine, S.; Szanto, T.; Hamer-Rogotner, S.; Dym, O.; Frolow, F.; Gordon, D.; Panyi, G.; Gurevitz, M.; et al. Pore-modulating toxins exploit inherent slow inactivation to block K$^+$ channels. *Proc. Natl. Acad. Sci. USA* **2019**, *116*, 18700–18709. [CrossRef]

61. Dave, K.; Lahiry, A. Conotoxins: Review and docking studies to determine potentials of conotoxin as an anticancer drug molecule. *Curr. Top. Med. Chem.* **2012**, *12*, 845–851. [CrossRef]

62. Puillandre, N.; Duda, T.F.; Meyer, C.; Olivera, B.M.; Bouchet, P. One, four or 100 genera? A new classification of the cone snails. *J. Molluscan Stud.* **2015**, *81*, 1–23. [CrossRef]

63. Dutertre, S.; Jin, A.H.; Vetter, I.; Hamilton, B.; Sunagar, K.; Lavergne, V.; Dutertre, V.; Fry, B.G.; Antunes, A.; Venter, D.J.; et al. Evolution of separate predation- and defence-evoked venoms in carnivorous cone snails. *Nat. Commun.* **2014**, *5*, 3521. [CrossRef]

64. Morales Duque, H.; Campos Dias, S.; Franco, O.L. Structural and Functional Analyses of Cone Snail Toxins. *Mar. Drugs* **2019**, *17*, 370. [CrossRef] [PubMed]

65. Olivera, B.M.; Raghuraman, S.; Schmidt, E.W.; Safavi-Hemami, H. Linking neuroethology to the chemical biology of natural products: Interactions between cone snails and their fish prey, a case study. *J. Comp. Physiol. A Neuroethol. Sens. Neural Behav. Physiol.* **2017**, *203*, 717–735. [CrossRef] [PubMed]

66. Teichert, R.W.; Schmidt, E.W.; Olivera, B.M. Constellation pharmacology: A new paradigm for drug discovery. *Annu. Rev. Pharmacol. Toxicol.* **2015**, *55*, 573–589. [CrossRef] [PubMed]

67. Han, T.S.; Teichert, R.W.; Olivera, B.M.; Bulaj, G. Conus venoms—A rich source of peptide-based therapeutics. *Curr. Pharm. Des.* **2008**, *14*, 2462–2479. [CrossRef]

68. Jin, A.H.; Muttenthaler, M.; Dutertre, S.; Himaya, S.W.A.; Kaas, Q.; Craik, D.J.; Lewis, R.J.; Alewood, P.F. Conotoxins: Chemistry and Biology. *Chem. Rev.* **2019**, *119*, 11510–11549. [CrossRef]

69. Lavergne, V.; Harliwong, I.; Jones, A.; Miller, D.; Taft, R.J.; Alewood, P.F. Optimized deep-targeted proteotranscriptomic profiling reveals unexplored Conus toxin diversity and novel cysteine frameworks. *Proc. Natl. Acad. Sci. USA* **2015**, *112*, E3782–E3791. [CrossRef]

70. Buczek, O.; Bulaj, G.; Olivera, B.M. Conotoxins and the posttranslational modification of secreted gene products. *Cell. Mol. Life Sci.* **2005**, *62*, 3067–3079. [CrossRef]

71. Kaas, Q.; Westermann, J.C.; Halai, R.; Wang, C.K.; Craik, D.J. ConoServer, a database for conopeptide sequences and structures. *Bioinformatics* **2008**, *24*, 445–446. [CrossRef]

72. Terlau, H.; Shon, K.J.; Grilley, M.; Stocker, M.; Stuhmer, W.; Olivera, B.M. Strategy for rapid immobilization of prey by a fish-hunting marine snail. *Nature* **1996**, *381*, 148–151. [CrossRef]

73. Tabakmakher, V.M.; Krylov, N.A.; Kuzmenkov, A.I.; Efremov, R.G.; Vassilevski, A.A. Kalium 2.0, a comprehensive database of polypeptide ligands of potassium channels. *Sci. Data* **2019**, *6*, 73. [CrossRef]

74. Massilia, G.R.; Eliseo, T.; Grolleau, F.; Lapied, B.; Barbier, J.; Bournaud, R.; Molgo, J.; Cicero, D.O.; Paci, M.; Schinina, M.E.; et al. Contryphan-Vn: A modulator of Ca^{2+}-dependent K^+ channels. *Biochem. Biophys. Res. Commun.* **2003**, *303*, 238–246. [CrossRef]

75. Scanlon, M.J.; Naranjo, D.; Thomas, L.; Alewood, P.F.; Lewis, R.J.; Craik, D.J. Solution structure and proposed binding mechanism of a novel potassium channel toxin kappa-conotoxin PVIIA. *Structure* **1997**, *5*, 1585–1597. [CrossRef]

76. Imperial, J.S.; Bansal, P.S.; Alewood, P.F.; Daly, N.L.; Craik, D.J.; Sporning, A.; Terlau, H.; Lopez-Vera, E.; Bandyopadhyay, P.K.; Olivera, B.M. A novel conotoxin inhibitor of Kv1.6 channel and nAChR subtypes defines a new superfamily of conotoxins. *Biochemistry* **2006**, *45*, 8331–8340. [CrossRef] [PubMed]

77. Ferber, M.; Al-Sabi, A.; Stocker, M.; Olivera, B.M.; Terlau, H. Identification of a mammalian target of kappaM-conotoxin RIIIK. *Toxicon* **2004**, *43*, 915–921. [CrossRef] [PubMed]

78. Cruz, L.J.; Gray, W.R.; Olivera, B.M.; Zeikus, R.D.; Kerr, L.; Yoshikami, D.; Moczydlowski, E. Conus geographus toxins that discriminate between neuronal and muscle sodium channels. *J. Biol. Chem.* **1985**, *260*, 9280–9288.

79. Ferber, M.; Sporning, A.; Jeserich, G.; DeLaCruz, R.; Watkins, M.; Olivera, B.M.; Terlau, H. A novel conus peptide ligand for K^+ channels. *J. Biol. Chem.* **2003**, *278*, 2177–2183. [CrossRef]

80. Chen, P.; Dendorfer, A.; Finol-Urdaneta, R.K.; Terlau, H.; Olivera, B.M. Biochemical characterization of kappaM-RIIIJ, a Kv1.2 channel blocker: Evaluation of cardioprotective effects of kappaM-conotoxins. *J. Biol. Chem.* **2010**, *285*, 14882–14889. [CrossRef]

81. Verdier, L.; Al-Sabi, A.; Rivier, J.E.; Olivera, B.M.; Terlau, H.; Carlomagno, T. Identification of a novel pharmacophore for peptide toxins interacting with K^+ channels. *J. Biol. Chem.* **2005**, *280*, 21246–21255. [CrossRef]

82. Cordeiro, S.; Finol-Urdaneta, R.K.; Kopfer, D.; Markushina, A.; Song, J.; French, R.J.; Kopec, W.; de Groot, B.L.; Giacobassi, M.J.; Leavitt, L.S.; et al. Conotoxin kappaM-RIIIJ, a tool targeting asymmetric heteromeric Kv1 channels. *Proc. Natl. Acad. Sci. USA* **2019**, *116*, 1059–1064. [CrossRef]

83. Giacobassi, M.J.; Leavitt, L.S.; Raghuraman, S.; Alluri, R.; Chase, K.; Finol-Urdaneta, R.K.; Terlau, H.; Teichert, R.W.; Olivera, B.M. An integrative approach to the facile functional classification of dorsal root ganglion neuronal subclasses. *Proc. Natl. Acad. Sci. USA* **2020**. [CrossRef]

84. Imperial, J.S.; Chen, P.; Sporning, A.; Terlau, H.; Daly, N.L.; Craik, D.J.; Alewood, P.F.; Olivera, B.M. Tyrosine-rich conopeptides affect voltage-gated K^+ channels. *J. Biol. Chem.* **2008**, *283*, 23026–23032. [CrossRef] [PubMed]

85. Kauferstein, S.; Huys, I.; Lamthanh, H.; Stocklin, R.; Sotto, F.; Menez, A.; Tytgat, J.; Mebs, D. A novel conotoxin inhibiting vertebrate voltage-sensitive potassium channels. *Toxicon* **2003**, *42*, 43–52. [CrossRef]

86. Dy, C.Y.; Buczek, P.; Imperial, J.S.; Bulaj, G.; Horvath, M.P. Structure of conkunitzin-S1, a neurotoxin and Kunitz-fold disulfide variant from cone snail. *Acta Crystallogr. D Biol. Crystallogr.* **2006**, *62 (Pt 9)*, 980–990. [CrossRef]

87. Korukottu, J.; Bayrhuber, M.; Montaville, P.; Vijayan, V.; Jung, Y.S.; Becker, S.; Zweckstetter, M. Fast high-resolution protein structure determination by using unassigned NMR data. *Angew. Chem. Int. Ed. Engl.* **2007**, *46*, 1176–1179. [CrossRef] [PubMed]

88. Cuello, L.G.; Jogini, V.; Cortes, D.M.; Perozo, E. Structural mechanism of C-type inactivation in K^+ channels. *Nature* **2010**, *466*, 203–208. [CrossRef] [PubMed]

89. Finol-Urdaneta, R.K. *Investigation of the Heterologous Expression of the Voltage Activated Potassium Channel Kv1.7*; George-August University: Goettingen, Germany, 2004.

90. Zhang, S.J.; Yang, X.M.; Liu, G.S.; Cohen, M.V.; Pemberton, K.; Downey, J.M. CGX-1051, a peptide from Conus snail venom, attenuates infarction in rabbit hearts when administered at reperfusion. *J. Cardiovasc. Pharmacol.* **2003**, *42*, 764–771. [CrossRef]

91. Lubbers, N.L.; Campbell, T.J.; Polakowski, J.S.; Bulaj, G.; Layer, R.T.; Moore, J.; Gross, G.J.; Cox, B.F. Postischemic administration of CGX-1051, a peptide from cone snail venom, reduces infarct size in both rat and dog models of myocardial ischemia and reperfusion. *J. Cardiovasc. Pharmacol.* **2005**, *46*, 141–146. [CrossRef]

92. Mahdavi, S.; Kuyucak, S. Why the Drosophila Shaker K^+ channel is not a good model for ligand binding to voltage-gated Kv1 channels. *Biochemistry* **2013**, *52*, 1631–1640. [CrossRef]

93. Tanaka, J.; Abe, J.; Futagi, Y. A case of late infantile ceroid lipofuscinosis–an electrophysiological follow-up study. *Hattatsu* **1987**, *19*, 415–419.

94. Aguilar, M.B.; Perez-Reyes, L.I.; Lopez, Z.; de la Cotera, E.P.; Falcon, A.; Ayala, C.; Galvan, M.; Salvador, C.; Escobar, L.I. Peptide sr11a from *Conus spurius* is a novel peptide blocker for Kv1 potassium channels. *Peptides* **2010**, *31*, 1287–1291. [CrossRef]

95. Mondal, S.; Babu, R.M.; Bhavna, R.; Ramakumar, S. In silico detection of binding mode of J-superfamily conotoxin pl14a with Kv1.6 channel. *Silico Biol* **2007**, *7*, 175–186.

96. Leipold, E.; Ullrich, F.; Thiele, M.; Tietze, A.A.; Terlau, H.; Imhof, D.; Heinemann, S.H. Subtype-specific block of voltage-gated K⁺ channels by mu-conopeptides. *Biochem. Biophys. Res. Commun.* **2017**, *482*, 1135–1140. [CrossRef] [PubMed]

97. Finol-Urdaneta, R.K.; McArthur, J.R.; Korkosh, V.S.; Huang, S.; McMaster, D.; Glavica, R.; Tikhonov, D.B.; Zhorov, B.S.; French, R.J. Extremely Potent Block of Bacterial Voltage-Gated Sodium Channels by micro-Conotoxin PIIIA. *Mar. Drugs* **2019**, *17*, 510. [CrossRef]

98. Kaufmann, D.; Tietze, A.A.; Tietze, D. In Silico Analysis of the Subtype Selective Blockage of KCNA Ion Channels through the micro-Conotoxins PIIIA, SIIIA, and GIIIA. *Mar. Drugs* **2019**, *17*, 180. [CrossRef]

99. Imperial, J.S.; Cabang, A.B.; Song, J.; Raghuraman, S.; Gajewiak, J.; Watkins, M.; Showers-Corneli, P.; Fedosov, A.; Concepcion, G.P.; Terlau, H.; et al. A family of excitatory peptide toxins from venomous crassispirine snails: Using Constellation Pharmacology to assess bioactivity. *Toxicon* **2014**, *89*, 45–54. [CrossRef] [PubMed]

100. Honma, T.; Shiomi, K. Peptide toxins in sea anemones: Structural and functional aspects. *Mar. Biotechnol. (N. Y.)* **2006**, *8*, 1–10. [CrossRef] [PubMed]

101. Kuyucak, S.; Norton, R.S. Computational approaches for designing potent and selective analogs of peptide toxins as novel therapeutics. *Future Med. Chem.* **2014**, *6*, 1645–1658. [CrossRef]

102. Prentis, P.J.; Pavasovic, A.; Norton, R.S. Sea Anemones: Quiet Achievers in the Field of Peptide Toxins. *Toxins (Basel)* **2018**, *10*, 36. [CrossRef]

103. Madio, B.; King, G.F.; Undheim, E.A.B. Sea Anemone Toxins: A Structural Overview. *Mar. Drugs* **2019**, *17*, 325. [CrossRef]

104. Gasparini, S.; Gilquin, B.; Menez, A. Comparison of sea anemone and scorpion toxins binding to Kv1 channels: An example of convergent evolution. *Toxicon* **2004**, *43*, 901–908. [CrossRef]

105. Mouhat, S.; Jouirou, B.; Mosbah, A.; De Waard, M.; Sabatier, J.M. Diversity of folds in animal toxins acting on ion channels. *Biochem. J.* **2004**, *378 (Pt 3)*, 717–726. [CrossRef]

106. Kalman, K.; Pennington, M.W.; Lanigan, M.D.; Nguyen, A.; Rauer, H.; Mahnir, V.; Paschetto, K.; Kem, W.R.; Grissmer, S.; Gutman, G.A.; et al. ShK-Dap22, a potent Kv1.3-specific immunosuppressive polypeptide. *J. Biol. Chem.* **1998**, *273*, 32697–32707. [CrossRef] [PubMed]

107. Pennington, M.W.; Mahnir, V.M.; Khaytin, I.; Zaydenberg, I.; Byrnes, M.E.; Kem, W.R. An essential binding surface for ShK toxin interaction with rat brain potassium channels. *Biochemistry* **1996**, *35*, 16407–16411. [CrossRef] [PubMed]

108. Minagawa, S.; Ishida, M.; Nagashima, Y.; Shiomi, K. Primary structure of a potassium channel toxin from the sea anemone *Actinia equina*. *FEBS Lett.* **1998**, *427*, 149–151. [CrossRef]

109. Hasegawa, Y.; Honma, T.; Nagai, H.; Ishida, M.; Nagashima, Y.; Shiomi, K. Isolation and cDNA cloning of a potassium channel peptide toxin from the sea anemone *Anemonia erythraea*. *Toxicon* **2006**, *48*, 536–542. [CrossRef] [PubMed]

110. Orts, D.J.; Moran, Y.; Cologna, C.T.; Peigneur, S.; Madio, B.; Praher, D.; Quinton, L.; De Pauw, E.; Bicudo, J.E.; Tytgat, J.; et al. BcsTx3 is a founder of a novel sea anemone toxin family of potassium channel blocker. *FEBS J.* **2013**, *280*, 4839–4852. [CrossRef] [PubMed]

111. Schweitz, H.; Bruhn, T.; Guillemare, E.; Moinier, D.; Lancelin, J.M.; Beress, L.; Lazdunski, M. Kalicludines and kaliseptine. Two different classes of sea anemone toxins for voltage sensitive K⁺ channels. *J. Biol. Chem.* **1995**, *270*, 25121–25126. [CrossRef]

112. Cotton, J.; Crest, M.; Bouet, F.; Alessandri, N.; Gola, M.; Forest, E.; Karlsson, E.; Castaneda, O.; Harvey, A.L.; Vita, C.; et al. A potassium-channel toxin from the sea anemone *Bunodosoma granulifera*, an inhibitor for Kv1 channels. Revision of the amino acid sequence, disulfide-bridge assignment, chemical synthesis, and biological activity. *Eur. J. Biochem.* **1997**, *244*, 192–202. [CrossRef]

113. Racape, J.; Lecoq, A.; Romi-Lebrun, R.; Liu, J.; Kohler, M.; Garcia, M.L.; Menez, A.; Gasparini, S. Characterization of a novel radiolabeled peptide selective for a subpopulation of voltage-gated potassium channels in mammalian brain. *J. Biol. Chem.* **2002**, *277*, 3886–3893. [CrossRef]

114. Gendeh, G.S.; Young, L.C.; de Medeiros, C.L.; Jeyaseelan, K.; Harvey, A.L.; Chung, M.C. A new potassium channel toxin from the sea anemone *Heteractis magnifica*: Isolation, cDNA cloning, and functional expression. *Biochemistry* **1997**, *36*, 11461–11471. [CrossRef]

115. Zhao, Y.; Huang, J.; Yuan, X.; Peng, B.; Liu, W.; Han, S.; He, X. Toxins Targeting the Kv1.3 Channel: Potential Immunomodulators for Autoimmune Diseases. *Toxins (Basel)* **2015**, *7*, 1749–1764. [CrossRef] [PubMed]

116. Diochot, S.; Lazdunski, M. Sea anemone toxins affecting potassium channels. *Prog. Mol. Subcell Biol.* **2009**, *46*, 99–122. [PubMed]

117. Honma, T.; Kawahata, S.; Ishida, M.; Nagai, H.; Nagashima, Y.; Shiomi, K. Novel peptide toxins from the sea anemone *Stichodactyla haddoni*. *Peptides* **2008**, *29*, 536–544. [CrossRef] [PubMed]

118. Diochot, S.; Loret, E.; Bruhn, T.; Beress, L.; Lazdunski, M. APETx1, a new toxin from the sea anemone *Anthopleura elegantissima*, blocks voltage-gated human ether-a-go-go-related gene potassium channels. *Mol. Pharmacol.* **2003**, *64*, 59–69. [CrossRef]

119. Rodriguez, A.A.; Garateix, A.; Salceda, E.; Peigneur, S.; Zaharenko, A.J.; Pons, T.; Santos, Y.; Arreguin, R.; Standker, L.; Forssmann, W.G.; et al. PhcrTx2, a New Crab-Paralyzing Peptide Toxin from the Sea Anemone *Phymanthus crucifer*. *Toxins (Basel)* **2018**, *10*, 72. [CrossRef]

120. Rodriguez, A.A.; Salceda, E.; Garateix, A.G.; Zaharenko, A.J.; Peigneur, S.; Lopez, O.; Pons, T.; Richardson, M.; Diaz, M.; Hernandez, Y.; et al. A novel sea anemone peptide that inhibits acid-sensing ion channels. *Peptides* **2014**, *53*, 3–12. [CrossRef]

121. DJ, B.O.; Peigneur, S.; Silva-Goncalves, L.C.; Arcisio-Miranda, M.; Je, P.W.B.; Tytgat, J. AbeTx1 Is a Novel Sea Anemone Toxin with a Dual Mechanism of Action on Shaker-Type K$^+$ Channels Activation. *Mar. Drugs* **2018**, *16*.

122. Chagot, B.; Escoubas, P.; Villegas, E.; Bernard, C.; Ferrat, G.; Corzo, G.; Lazdunski, M.; Darbon, H. Solution structure of Phrixotoxin 1, a specific peptide inhibitor of Kv4 potassium channels from the venom of the theraphosid spider *Phrixotrichus auratus*. *Protein Sci.* **2004**, *13*, 1197–1208. [CrossRef]

123. Driscoll, P.C.; Gronenborn, A.M.; Beress, L.; Clore, G.M. Determination of the three-dimensional solution structure of the antihypertensive and antiviral protein BDS-I from the sea anemone *Anemonia sulcata*: A study using nuclear magnetic resonance and hybrid distance geometry-dynamical simulated annealing. *Biochemistry* **1989**, *28*, 2188–2198. [CrossRef]

124. Rauer, H.; Pennington, M.; Cahalan, M.; Chandy, K.G. Structural conservation of the pores of calcium-activated and voltage-gated potassium channels determined by a sea anemone toxin. *J. Biol. Chem.* **1999**, *274*, 21885–21892. [CrossRef]

125. Castaneda, O.; Sotolongo, V.; Amor, A.M.; Stocklin, R.; Anderson, A.J.; Harvey, A.L.; Engstrom, A.; Wernstedt, C.; Karlsson, E. Characterization of a potassium channel toxin from the Caribbean Sea anemone *Stichodactyla helianthus*. *Toxicon* **1995**, *33*, 603–613. [CrossRef]

126. Pennington, M.W.; Mahnir, V.M.; Krafte, D.S.; Zaydenberg, I.; Byrnes, M.E.; Khaytin, I.; Crowley, K.; Kem, W.R. Identification of three separate binding sites on SHK toxin, a potent inhibitor of voltage-dependent potassium channels in human T-lymphocytes and rat brain. *Biochem. Biophys. Res. Commun.* **1996**, *219*, 696–701. [CrossRef] [PubMed]

127. Chang, S.C.; Huq, R.; Chhabra, S.; Beeton, C.; Pennington, M.W.; Smith, B.J.; Norton, R.S. N-Terminally extended analogues of the K$^+$ channel toxin from Stichodactyla helianthus as potent and selective blockers of the voltage-gated potassium channel Kv1.3. *FEBS J.* **2015**, *282*, 2247–2259. [CrossRef] [PubMed]

128. Murray, J.K.; Qian, Y.X.; Liu, B.; Elliott, R.; Aral, J.; Park, C.; Zhang, X.; Stenkilsson, M.; Salyers, K.; Rose, M.; et al. Pharmaceutical Optimization of Peptide Toxins for Ion Channel Targets: Potent, Selective, and Long-Lived Antagonists of Kv1.3. *J. Med. Chem.* **2015**, *58*, 6784–6802. [CrossRef]

129. Yan, L.; Herrington, J.; Goldberg, E.; Dulski, P.M.; Bugianesi, R.M.; Slaughter, R.S.; Banerjee, P.; Brochu, R.M.; Priest, B.T.; Kaczorowski, G.J.; et al. *Stichodactyla helianthus* peptide, a pharmacological tool for studying Kv3.2 channels. *Mol. Pharmacol.* **2005**, *67*, 1513–1521. [CrossRef]

130. Garcia-Fernandez, R.; Peigneur, S.; Pons, T.; Alvarez, C.; Gonzalez, L.; Chavez, M.A.; Tytgat, J. The Kunitz-Type Protein ShPI-1 Inhibits Serine Proteases and Voltage-Gated Potassium Channels. *Toxins (Basel)* **2016**, *8*, 110. [CrossRef]

131. Chi, V.; Pennington, M.W.; Norton, R.S.; Tarcha, E.J.; Londono, L.M.; Sims-Fahey, B.; Upadhyay, S.K.; Lakey, J.T.; Iadonato, S.; Wulff, H.; et al. Development of a sea anemone toxin as an immunomodulator for therapy of autoimmune diseases. *Toxicon* **2012**, *59*, 529–546. [CrossRef]

132. Pennington, M.W.; Harunur Rashid, M.; Tajhya, R.B.; Beeton, C.; Kuyucak, S.; Norton, R.S. A C-terminally amidated analogue of ShK is a potent and selective blocker of the voltage-gated potassium channel Kv1.3. *FEBS Lett.* **2012**, *586*, 3996–4001. [CrossRef]

133. Gilquin, B.; Braud, S.; Eriksson, M.A.; Roux, B.; Bailey, T.D.; Priest, B.T.; Garcia, M.L.; Menez, A.; Gasparini, S. A variable residue in the pore of Kv1 channels is critical for the high affinity of blockers from sea anemones and scorpions. *J. Biol. Chem.* **2005**, *280*, 27093–27102. [CrossRef]

134. Alessandri-Haber, N.; Lecoq, A.; Gasparini, S.; Grangier-Macmath, G.; Jacquet, G.; Harvey, A.L.; de Medeiros, C.; Rowan, E.G.; Gola, M.; Menez, A.; et al. Mapping the functional anatomy of BgK on Kv1.1, Kv1.2, and Kv1.3. Clues to design analogs with enhanced selectivity. *J. Biol. Chem.* **1999**, *274*, 35653–35661. [CrossRef]

135. Beraud, E.; Viola, A.; Regaya, I.; Confort-Gouny, S.; Siaud, P.; Ibarrola, D.; Le Fur, Y.; Barbaria, J.; Pellissier, J.F.; Sabatier, J.M.; et al. Block of neural Kv1.1 potassium channels for neuroinflammatory disease therapy. *Ann. Neurol.* **2006**, *60*, 586–596. [CrossRef] [PubMed]

136. Peigneur, S.; Billen, B.; Derua, R.; Waelkens, E.; Debaveye, S.; Beress, L.; Tytgat, J. A bifunctional sea anemone peptide with Kunitz type protease and potassium channel inhibiting properties. *Biochem. Pharmacol.* **2011**, *82*, 81–90. [CrossRef] [PubMed]

137. Mourao, C.B.; Schwartz, E.F. Protease inhibitors from marine venomous animals and their counterparts in terrestrial venomous animals. *Mar. Drugs* **2013**, *11*, 2069–2112. [CrossRef] [PubMed]

138. Ganz, T. Defensins: Antimicrobial peptides of vertebrates. *Comptes Rendus Biol.* **2004**, *327*, 539–549. [CrossRef] [PubMed]

139. Chagot, B.; Escoubas, P.; Diochot, S.; Bernard, C.; Lazdunski, M.; Darbon, H. Solution structure of APETx2, a specific peptide inhibitor of ASIC3 proton-gated channels. *Protein Sci.* **2005**, *14*, 2003–2010. [CrossRef] [PubMed]

140. Smith, J.J.; Blumenthal, K.M. Site-3 sea anemone toxins: Molecular probes of gating mechanisms in voltage-dependent sodium channels. *Toxicon* **2007**, *49*, 159–170. [CrossRef]

141. Beress, L.D.; Doppelfeld, I.S.; Etschenberg, E.; Graf, E.; Henschen, A.; Zwick, J. Polypeptides, Process for Their Preparation, and Their Use as Hypotensive Active Compounds. Patent No. DE3324689, 17 January 1985.

142. Liu, P.; Jo, S.; Bean, B.P. Modulation of neuronal sodium channels by the sea anemone peptide BDS-I. *J. Neurophysiol.* **2012**, *107*, 3155–3167. [CrossRef]

143. Moreels, L.; Peigneur, S.; Galan, D.T.; De Pauw, E.; Beress, L.; Waelkens, E.; Pardo, L.A.; Quinton, L.; Tytgat, J. APETx4, a Novel Sea Anemone Toxin and a Modulator of the Cancer-Relevant Potassium Channel Kv10.1. *Mar. Drugs* **2017**, *15*, 287. [CrossRef]

144. Daly, M.; Chaudhuri, A.; Gusmao, L.; Rodriguez, E. Phylogenetic relationships among sea anemones (Cnidaria: Anthozoa: Actiniaria). *Mol. Phylogenet. Evol.* **2008**, *48*, 292–301. [CrossRef]

145. Daly, N.L.; Craik, D.J. Bioactive cystine knot proteins. *Curr. Opin. Chem. Biol.* **2011**, *15*, 362–368. [CrossRef]

146. Konoki, K.; Suga, Y.; Fuwa, H.; Yotsu-Yamashita, M.; Sasaki, M. Evaluation of gambierol and its analogs for their inhibition of human Kv1.2 and cytotoxicity. *Bioorg. Med. Chem. Lett.* **2015**, *25*, 514–518. [CrossRef] [PubMed]

147. Lewis, R.J. Ciguatera: Australian perspectives on a global problem. *Toxicon* **2006**, *48*, 799–809. [CrossRef] [PubMed]

148. Cuypers, E.; Abdel-Mottaleb, Y.; Kopljar, I.; Rainier, J.D.; Raes, A.L.; Snyders, D.J.; Tytgat, J. Gambierol, a toxin produced by the dinoflagellate *Gambierdiscus toxicus*, is a potent blocker of voltage-gated potassium channels. *Toxicon* **2008**, *51*, 974–983. [CrossRef] [PubMed]

149. Kopljar, I.; Labro, A.J.; Cuypers, E.; Johnson, H.W.; Rainier, J.D.; Tytgat, J.; Snyders, D.J. A polyether biotoxin binding site on the lipid-exposed face of the pore domain of Kv channels revealed by the marine toxin gambierol. *Proc. Natl. Acad. Sci. USA* **2009**, *106*, 9896–9901. [CrossRef] [PubMed]

150. Fan, Z.; Ji, X.; Fu, M.; Zhang, W.; Zhang, D.; Xiao, Z. Electrostatic interaction between inactivation ball and T1-S1 linker region of Kv1.4 channel. *Biochim. Biophys. Acta* **2012**, *1818*, 55–63. [CrossRef] [PubMed]

151. Tang, Y.H.; Liang, T.T.; Fan, T.T.; Keen, L.J.; Zhang, X.D.; Xu, L.; Zhao, Q.; Zeng, R.; Han, B.N. Neo-debromoaplysiatoxin C, with new structural rearrangement, derived from debromoaplysiatoxin. *Nat. Prod. Res.* **2019**, 1–6. [CrossRef]

152. Nokura, Y.; Araki, Y.; Nakazaki, A.; Nishikawa, T. Synthetic Route to Oscillatoxin D and Its Analogues. *Org. Lett.* **2017**, *19*, 5992–5995. [CrossRef]

153. Dias, L.C.; Polo, E.C. Nhatrangin A: Total Syntheses of the Proposed Structure and Six of Its Diastereoisomers. *J. Org. Chem.* **2017**, *82*, 4072–4112. [CrossRef]

154. Fan, T.T.; Zhang, H.H.; Tang, Y.H.; Zhang, F.Z.; Han, B.N. Two New Neo-debromoaplysiatoxins-A Pair of Stereoisomers Exhibiting Potent Kv1.5 Ion Channel Inhibition Activities. *Mar. Drugs* **2019**, *17*, 652. [CrossRef]

155. Feng, J.; Wang, Z.; Li, G.R.; Nattel, S. Effects of class III antiarrhythmic drugs on transient outward and ultra-rapid delayed rectifier currents in human atrial myocytes. *J. Pharmacol. Exp. Ther.* **1997**, *281*, 384–392.

156. Hurst, R.S.; Kavanaugh, M.P.; Yakel, J.; Adelman, J.P.; North, R.A. Cooperative interactions among subunits of a voltage-dependent potassium channel. Evidence from expression of concatenated cDNAs. *J. Biol. Chem.* **1992**, *267*, 23742–23745. [PubMed]

157. Hurst, R.S.; North, R.A.; Adelman, J.P. Potassium channel assembly from concatenated subunits: Effects of proline substitutions in S4 segments. *Recept. Channels* **1995**, *3*, 263–272. [PubMed]

158. Klein-Schwartz, W.; Stassinos, G.L.; Isbister, G.K. Treatment of sulfonylurea and insulin overdose. *Br. J. Clin. Pharmacol.* **2016**, *81*, 496–504. [CrossRef] [PubMed]

159. Beeton, C.; Pennington, M.W.; Norton, R.S. Analogs of the sea anemone potassium channel blocker ShK for the treatment of autoimmune diseases. *Inflamm. Allergy Drug Targets* **2011**, *10*, 313–321. [CrossRef]

160. Pennington, M.W.; Beeton, C.; Galea, C.A.; Smith, B.J.; Chi, V.; Monaghan, K.P.; Garcia, A.; Rangaraju, S.; Giuffrida, A.; Plank, D.; et al. Engineering a stable and selective peptide blocker of the Kv1.3 channel in T lymphocytes. *Mol. Pharmacol.* **2009**, *75*, 762–773. [CrossRef]

161. Rosano, G.L.; Ceccarelli, E.A. Recombinant protein expression in *Escherichia coli*: Advances and challenges. *Front. Microbiol.* **2014**, *5*, 172. [CrossRef]

162. Stefan, A.; Ceccarelli, A.; Conte, E.; Monton Silva, A.; Hochkoeppler, A. The multifaceted benefits of protein co-expression in *Escherichia coli*. *J. Vis. Exp.* **2015**. [CrossRef]

163. Fahnert, B. Using folding promoting agents in recombinant protein production: A review. *Methods Mol. Biol.* **2012**, *824*, 3–36.

164. Khan, K.H. Gene expression in Mammalian cells and its applications. *Adv. Pharm. Bull.* **2013**, *3*, 257–263.

165. Luna-Ramirez, K.; Csoti, A.; McArthur, J.R.; Chin, Y.K.Y.; Anangi, R.; Najera, R.D.C.; Possani, L.D.; King, G.F.; Panyi, G.; Yu, H.; et al. Structural basis of the potency and selectivity of Urotoxin, a potent Kv1 blocker from scorpion venom. *Biochem. Pharmacol.* **2020**, *174*, 113782. [CrossRef]

166. Baneyx, F.; Mujacic, M. Recombinant protein folding and misfolding in Escherichia coli. *Nat. Biotechnol.* **2004**, *22*, 1399–1408. [CrossRef] [PubMed]

167. Denks, K.; Vogt, A.; Sachelaru, I.; Petriman, N.A.; Kudva, R.; Koch, H.G. The Sec translocon mediated protein transport in prokaryotes and eukaryotes. *Mol. Membr. Biol.* **2014**, *31*, 58–84. [CrossRef] [PubMed]

168. Lindequist, U. Marine-Derived Pharmaceuticals—Challenges and Opportunities. *Biomol. Ther. (Seoul)* **2016**, *24*, 561–571. [CrossRef] [PubMed]

169. Alves, C.; Silva, J.; Pinteus, S.; Gaspar, H.; Alpoim, M.C.; Botana, L.M.; Pedrosa, R. From Marine Origin to Therapeutics: The Antitumor Potential of Marine Algae-Derived Compounds. *Front. Pharmacol.* **2018**, *9*, 777. [CrossRef]

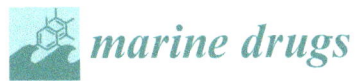

Review

Synthetic Approaches to Zetekitoxin AB, a Potent Voltage-Gated Sodium Channel Inhibitor

Kanna Adachi, Hayate Ishizuka, Minami Odagi * and Kazuo Nagasawa *

Department of Biotechnology and Life Science, Tokyo University of Agriculture and Technology (TUAT), 2-24-16, Naka-cho, Koganei city, Tokyo 184-8588, Japan; s175364y@st.go.tuat.ac.jp (K.A.); s189783w@st.go.tuat.ac.jp (H.I.)
* Correspondence: odagi@cc.tuat.ac.jp(M.O.); knaga@cc.tuat.ac.jp (K.N.)

Received: 7 December 2019; Accepted: 24 December 2019; Published: 26 December 2019

Abstract: Voltage-gated sodium channels (Na_Vs) are membrane proteins that are involved in the generation and propagation of action potentials in neurons. Recently, the structure of a complex made of a tetrodotoxin-sensitive (TTX-s) Na_V subtype with saxitoxin (STX), a shellfish toxin, was determined. STX potently inhibits TTX-s Na_V, and is used as a biological tool to investigate the function of Na_Vs. More than 50 analogs of STX have been isolated from nature. Among them, zetekitoxin AB (ZTX) has a distinctive chemical structure, and is the most potent inhibitor of Na_Vs, including tetrodotoxin-resistant (TTX-r) Na_V. Despite intensive synthetic studies, total synthesis of ZTX has not yet been achieved. Here, we review recent efforts directed toward the total synthesis of ZTX, including syntheses of 11-saxitoxinethanoic acid (SEA), which is considered a useful synthetic model for ZTX, since it contains a key carbon–carbon bond at the C11 position.

Keywords: saxitoxin; zetekitoxin AB; voltage-gated sodium channel; guanidine alkaloid

---

1. Introduction

1.1. Voltage-Gated Sodium Channel Isoforms

Voltage-gated sodium channels (Na_Vs) are membrane proteins involved in neuronal excitation and transmission [1]. Ten subtypes, Na_V1.1–1.9 and Na_VX, have been identified based on sequence determination (Table 1) [2]. These subtypes can be grouped into two types depending upon their sensitivity to the pufferfish toxin, tetrodotoxin (TTX) [3–7]: tetrodotoxin-sensitive Na_Vs (TTX-s Na_Vs 1.1–1.4, 1.6, and 1.7) are significantly inhibited by TTX, while tetrodotoxin-resistant Na_Vs (TTX-r Na_Vs 1.5, 1.8, 1.9) are not [8–23]. Subtype-selective modulators of Na_Vs are required for studies to establish the biological functions of these subtypes. Some of the subtypes are also considered to be potential drug targets; for example, Na_V1.7 and 1.8 are potential targets for pain treatment [24–29]. Therefore, there is great interest in the development of drugs targeting specific subtypes [30,31].

Table 1. Isoforms of a voltage-gated sodium channel (Na_V) and their classifications.

Na_V Isoform	Primary Locations	Related Diseases	TTX IC_{50} (nM)
TTX-sensitive			
$Na_V1.1$	CNS, PNS, heart	Epilepsy	5.9
$Na_V1.2$	CNS	Epilepsy	7.8
$Na_V1.3$	Embryonic CNS, injured DRG	Nerve injury	2.0
$Na_V1.4$	Skeletal muscle	Myotonia	4.5
$Na_V1.6$	CNS, PNS, SMCs, DRG	CNS disorders	3.8
$Na_V1.7$	PNS, DRG	Pain sensation	5.5
TTX-resistant			
$Na_V1.5$	Heart, embryonic CNS	Cardiac arrhythmias	1970
$Na_V1.8$	PNS, DRG	Pain sensation	1330
$Na_V1.9$	PNS, DRG	Pain sensation	59,600

TTX: tetrodotoxin; CNS: central nervous system; PNS: peripheral nervous system; DRG: dorsal root ganglion; SMCs: smooth muscle cells.

1.2. Saxitoxin As A Na_V Modulator

Saxitoxin (STX, **1**) is a guanidine alkaloid with potent and specific inhibitory activity towards Na_Vs (Figure 1) [32,33]. It has long been known as a shellfish toxin. In 1937, Sommer and co-workers found that toxin-free bivalves, including the dinoflagellate *Gonyaulax catenella*, became poisoned in seawater, and they revealed that the real producer of STX (**1**) is algae [34,35]. Then, STX (**1**) was first isolated from Alaska butter clams by Schantz's group in 1957 [36,37]. Rapport's group subsequently isolated the same toxin from the same shellfish, and named it saxitoxin [38]. Structural elucidation was troublesome. Initially, tri- or tetracyclic structures were proposed based upon the molecular formula and the presence of two guanidines as functional groups. Finally, the structure of STX (**1**) was independently determined by the two groups by means of X-ray analysis in 1975 [39,40]. STX (**1**) consists of ten carbons, seven nitrogens, and four oxygens, and all the carbons except for C11 are connected with heteroatoms. STX (**1**) contains five- and six-membered cyclic guanidines, which have different pKa values of 8.7 and 12.4, respectively; the five-membered one is less basic, presumably due to its less planar structure [41].

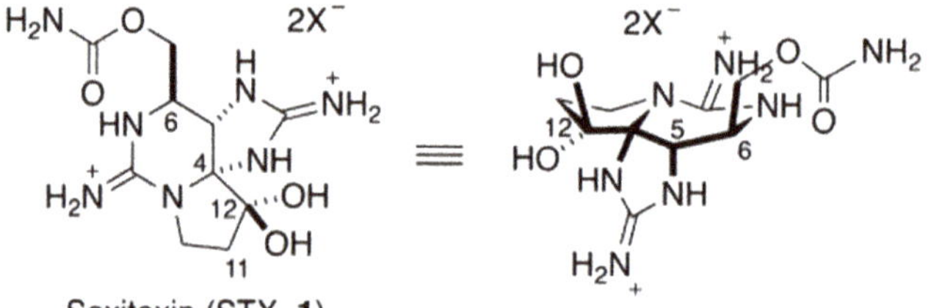

Figure 1. Structure of saxitoxin (STX, **1**).

STX (**1**) binds to the pore-forming region of the alpha-loop of Na_V and blocks the influx of sodium cation in a similar manner to tetrodotoxin (TTX) [42,43]. Recently, Yan's group determined the X-ray structure of the complexes of STX (**1**) with Na_VPas derived from American cockroach and human-derived $Na_V1.7$ by using cryoEM (Figure 2) [44,45]. They found that the carbamoyl group at C13 in STX (**1**) interacts with Gly1407 and Thr1409 in domain III, the two guanidines interact with Glu364 in domain I and Glu930 in domain II, and the geminal diol interacts with Asp1701 in domain IV. Interestingly, residues 1409 and 1410, located in the P2 loop of domain III in $Na_V1.7$, were mutated to Thr and Ile from Met and Asp, respectively, which may explain why STX (**1**) has a weaker affinity for $Na_V1.7$ compared with other subtypes (Met1409 and Asp1410 are conserved in the other subtypes of TTX-s) [46,47].

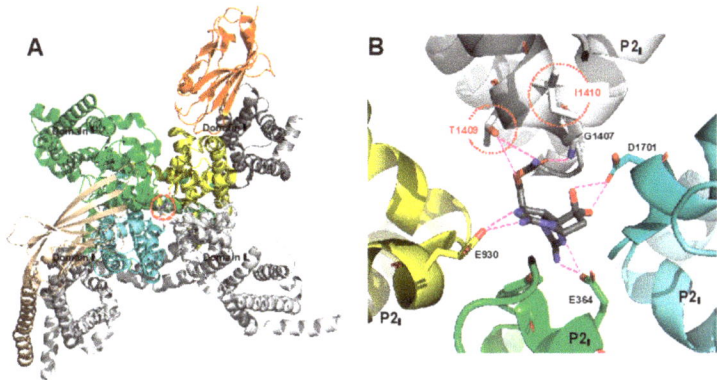

Figure 2. (**A**) Top view of the structure of the STX–Na$_V$1.7 complex. (**B**) Specific interactions in the STX–Na$_V$1.7 complex [45].

1.3. Natural Analogs of Saxitoxin, Including Zetekitoxin AB (ZTX)

To date, more than 50 kinds of natural analogs of saxitoxin have been reported, of which most are modified at N1 (R^1), C11 (i.e., R^2 and R^3), or C13 (R^4) in the common structure shown in Figure 3A [48]. For example, neosaxitoxin (neoSTX, **2**) is hydroxylated at N1, decarbamoylsaxitoxin (dcSTX, **3**) has a hydroxyl group at C13, and gonyautoxins I–III (GTX I–III, **5–7**, respectively) have a sulfate ester at C11; all of these analogs show similar Na$_V$-inhibitory activity to STX (**1**).

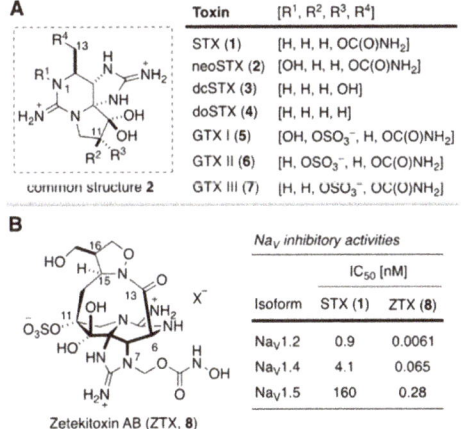

Figure 3. (**A**) Representative STX derivatives. (**B**) Structure and Na$_V$-inhibitory activities of zetekitoxin AB (**8**) [49].

Among the STX (**1**) derivatives, zetekitoxin AB (ZTX, **8**) has an unusual structure [49]. ZTX (**8**) was isolated from skin of the Panamanian dart-poison frog *Atelopus zeteki* in 1969 by Mosher and co-workers [50,51]. It has extremely potent Na$_V$-inhibitory activity (more than 600-fold greater than that of STX (**1**)), with IC$_{50}$ values of 6.1 pM, 65 pM, and 280 pM for Na$_V$1.2, Na$_V$1.4, and TTX-r subtype Na$_V$1.5, respectively [49]. Thus, there is great interest in the mode of action of ZTX (**8**), but studies are hampered by the fact that *Atelopus zeteki* is designated as an endangered species. Therefore, a chemical synthesis of ZTX (**8**) is needed. However, ZTX (**8**) contains a macrocyclic lactam structure in which isoxazolidine is bridged from C6 to C11, and an *N*-hydroxycarbamate is linked via a methylene group at N7 [49]. These structural features make ZTX (**8**) synthetically challenging. So far, several synthetic approaches have been reported, but a total synthesis of **8** has not yet been achieved.

1.4. Scope of This Review

Synthetic studies of STX (**1**) and its analogs have been extensive, and several total syntheses have been achieved [52–61], as recently reviewed by Du Bois [62]. Approaches for developing of subtype-selective modulators based on the STX structure have also been explored [25,47,63–65]. However, in this review, we focus on recent synthetic work related to ZTX (**8**). As described above, ZTX (**8**) has a characteristic macrolactam structure though C6 to C11 with an isoxazolidine ring system, and is structurally quite distinct from other STX analogs. To achieve total synthesis of ZTX (**8**), two key issues must be addressed: (i) carbon–carbon bond formation at the C11 position in the STX skeleton, and (ii) macrolactam formation of the carboxylic acid at C6 with isoxazolidine nitrogen (Figure 4). Regarding the first issue, the STX derivative 11-saxitoxinethanoic acid (SEA, **9**) has been used as a synthetic model for **8**, since it also has a carbon–carbon bond at the C11 position. As for the second issue, stereoselective synthesis of disubstituted isoxazolidine and oxidation to carboxylic acid at C13, followed by amide formation with the isoxazolidine, have been examined. First, we will consider recent progress in the total synthesis of SEA (**9**).

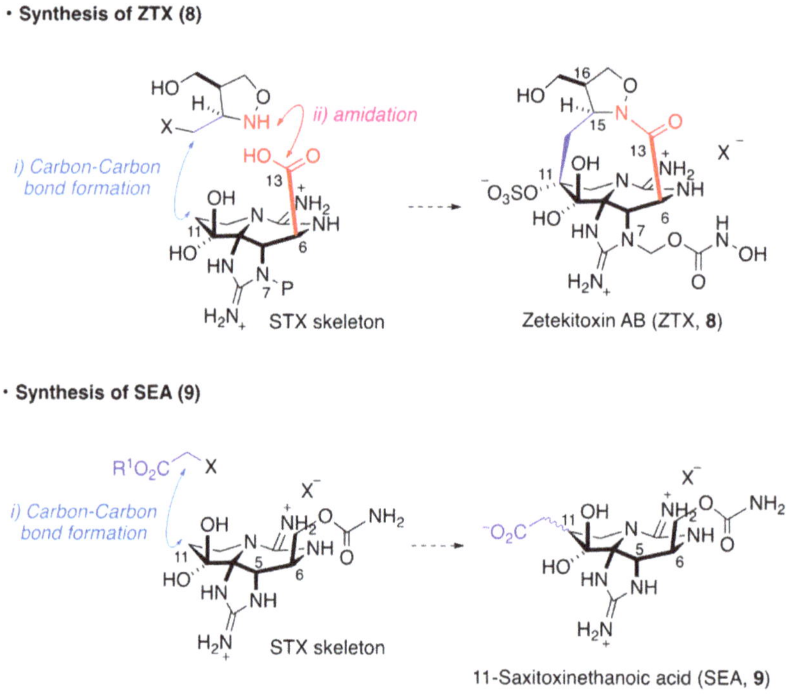

Figure 4. Key issues in the synthesis of ZTX (**8**) and 11-saxitoxinethanoic acid (SEA, **9**).

2. Development of Carbon–Carbon Linkage at C11 of STX, And Application to The Synthesis of 11-Saxitoxinethanoic Acid (SEA, 9)

The STX analog 11-saxitoxinethanoic acid (SEA, **9**) was isolated from *Atergatis floridus*, an Indo-Pacific crab from the family Xanthidae, by Onoue and co-workers (Figure 5) [66]. SEA (**9**) has an acetic acid moiety linked to C11 through a carbon–carbon bond, as seen in ZTX (**8**), and is regarded as a promising synthetic model compound for **8** in terms of construction of the carbon–carbon connection at C11.

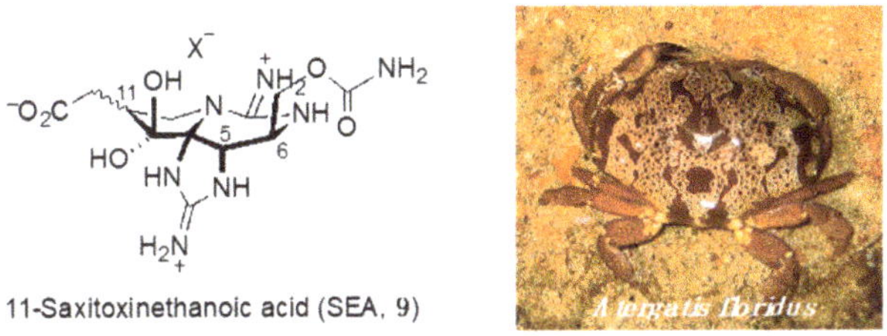

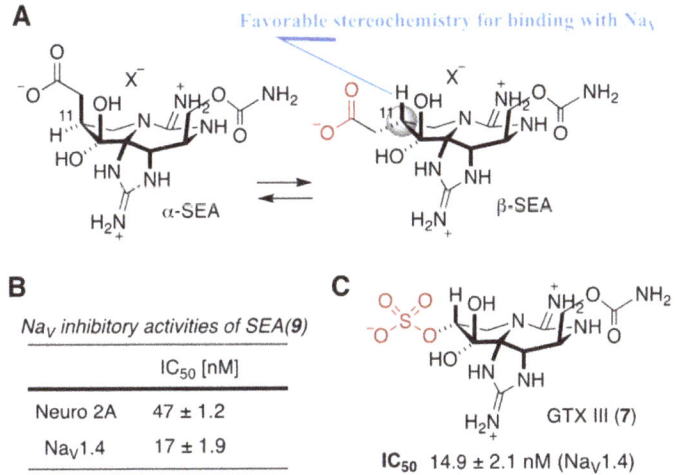

Figure 5. Structure of 11-saxitoxinethanoic acid (SEA, **9**) and illustration of the source crab species.

Recently, three total synthesis of SEA (**9**) were independently reported, including one by our group [67–69]. When **9** was first isolated, its toxicity to mice was reported to be 830 μmol/MU, which is similar to that of gonyautoxin II (GTX II, **6**) and one-third of that of STX (**1**), but no information about the Na$_V$-inhibitory activity was provided. After the synthesis of **9**, Du Bois and our group independently evaluated the Na$_V$-inhibitory activity of **9**. Nagasawa, Yotsu-Yamashita, and co-workers evaluated the Na$_V$-inhibitory activity of SEA (**9**) by utilizing neuroblastoma Neuro 2A cells, which is known to express Na$_V$1.2, 1.3, 1.4, and 1.7 [70], and found moderate inhibitory activity with an IC$_{50}$ value of 47.0 ± 1.2 nM (Figure 6B) [67]. Du Bois and co-workers evaluated the inhibitory activity of **9** against Na$_V$1.4, and found that SEA (**9**) showed similar inhibitory activity to gonyautoxin III (GTX III, **7**) (**9**: IC$_{50}$ = 17 ± 1.9 nM; GTX III (**7**): IC$_{50}$ = 14.9 ± 2.1 nM), even though it was a diastereomeric mixture of α:β = 3:1 at C11 (Figure 6A) [68]. They suggested that the β-form of **9** binds to Na$_V$ preferentially, and then the α-form of **9** isomerizes to the β-form, which shows a similar level of inhibitory activity to GTX III (**7**) (Figure 6C).

A

Favorable stereochemistry for binding with Na$_V$

α-SEA

β-SEA

B

Na$_V$ inhibitory activities of SEA(**9**)

	IC$_{50}$ [nM]
Neuro 2A	47 ± 1.2
Na$_V$1.4	17 ± 1.9

C

GTX III (**7**)

IC$_{50}$ 14.9 ± 2.1 nM (Na$_V$1.4)

Figure 6. (**A**) Isomerization of α-SEA to β-SEA. (**B**) Na$_V$-inhibitory activity of SEA (**9**) [69,70]. (**C**) Structure of GTX III (**7**) and IC$_{50}$ (Na$_V$1.4).

2.1. Carbon–Carbon Bond Formation at C11 by Mukaiyama Aldol Condensation Reaction, as Applied for The Synthesis of (+)-SEA by Nagasawa's Group

For the construction of a carbon–carbon bond at C11, Nagasawa and co-workers utilized ketone **10**, which was previously developed by their group [67], to install an acetic acid equivalent at C11. They firstly investigated the alkylation reaction of the enolate of ketone **10a** with alpha-halo-ethyl acetate. With various bases and halogens, the alkylation did not take place at all, and the starting ketone **10a** was recovered. Next, they investigated the Mukaiyama aldol reaction [71–73]. Thus, silyl enol ethers **11a** and **11b** were synthesized from the ketone by reaction with *tert*-butyldimethylsilyl chloride in the presence of NaHMDS as a base. Then, the Mukaiyama aldol reaction was examined with ethyl glyoxylate under various conditions. Lewis acids, such as $TiCl_4$ or BF_3 Et_2O [74,75], removed the *tert*-butoxycarbonyl (Boc) protecting group of guanidine, and no coupling products with ethyl glyoxylate were obtained. In the case of the fluoride anion agent Bu_4NF [76], the reaction did not proceed at all. On the other hand, with anhydrous tetrabutyl bisfluorotriphenylphosphine stannate, developed by Raimundo and co-workers [77], the coupling reaction with ethyl glyoxylate proceeded very well to afford the aldol-condensation product **12a** a 96% yield (Table 2). Aromatic aldehydes were tolerated, as well as aliphatic aldehydes, and the corresponding aldol condensation products **12a–i** were obtained with 42%–80% yield. This reaction afforded mixtures of regioisomers in ratios of 5:1 to >10:1.

Table 2. Substrate scope of the Mukaiyama aldol condensation reaction of **11a** and **11b** with aldehydes.

Entry.	SM	R^2	12 (E:Z) [a]	Yield (%)
1	11a	CO_2Et	**12a** (5:1)	96
2	11b	CO_2Et	**12b** (5:1)	85
3	11a	4-MeC_6H_4	**12c** (> 1:1)	45
4	11a	3-FC_6H_4	**12d** (> 10:1)	63
5	11a	4-ClC_6H_4	**12e** (> 10:1)	65
6	11a	$4\text{-NO}_2C_6H_4$	**12f** (6:1)	80
7	11a	2-Furyl	**12g** (> 10:1)	80
8	11a	C_6H_5	**12h** (> 10:1)	60
9	11b	C_6H_5	**12i** (E:Z) [a]	42

[a] Ration at C11 were determined by 1H NMR spectroscopy.

With the aldol condensation product **12b** in hand, Nagasawa and co-workers went on to achieve a total synthesis of (+)-SEA (**9**) for the first time (Scheme 1). Thus, selective reduction of the enone moiety in **12b** was carried out with L-selectride, and the protecting group of *tert*-butyldimethylsilyl (TBS) ether was removed with triethylamine trihydrofluoride (3HF-TEA). The resulting alcohol was reacted with trichloroisocyanate, followed by hydrolysis of the trichloroacetyl group with triethylamine in methanol to give carbamoyl **15**. After hydrolysis of ethyl ester in **15** with lithium hydroxide, the Boc group was removed with TFA to give (+)-SEA (**9**).

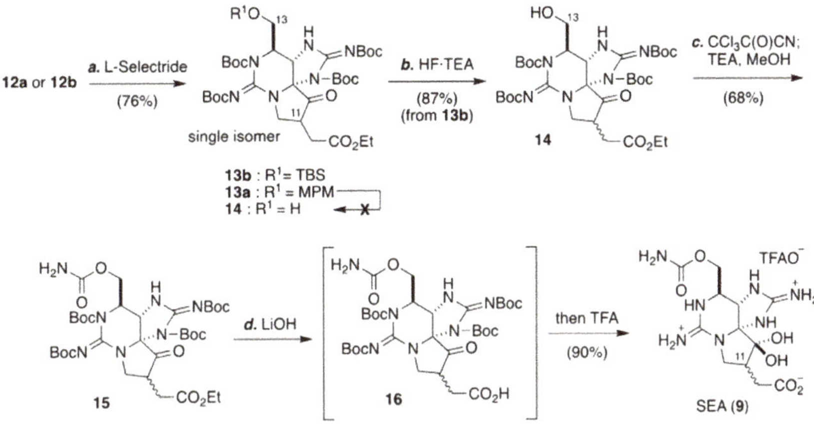

Scheme 1. Total synthesis of SEA (**9**) by Nagasawa's group.

2.2. Carbon–Carbon Bond Formation At C11 by Stille Coupling Reaction, As Applied for The Synthesis of (+)-SEA by Du Bois' Group

Another approach for the construction of the carbon–carbon bond at C11 in STX was explored by Du Bois and co-workers, who employed Stille coupling reaction conditions [68]. They firstly examined the coupling reaction of zinc enolate of ethyl acetate or the stannane enolate of ethyl acetate-type agents with vinyl halide **17**, which was prepared from **20**, developed by their group (Scheme 2), in the presence of palladium catalyst (Table 3, entries 1 and 2) [78–83]. Under the conditions examined, decomposition of the starting substrate was observed in the case of zinc agent, and no reaction occurred with the stannane agent. Then they examined the Stille coupling reaction, using vinyl stannane for the construction of the carbon–carbon bond at C11 [84]. A Stille coupling reaction of vinyl iodide **17** with tributyl(vinyl)tin was examined in the presence of a catalytic amount of Pd(PPh$_3$)$_4$, with CuI as an additive (a standard condition). Unfortunately, only a trace amount of the corresponding coupling product of **18c** was obtained (entry 3). Then, they changed vinyl stannane to cis-tributyl (2-ethoxyvinyl) tin, and included LiCl as an additional additive. Under these conditions, the corresponding coupling product **18d** was obtained with 67% yield (entry 4) [85,86]. Interestingly, poor reproducibility or low yield of the coupling reaction was observed when they used a highly oxidized vinyl stannane agent, tributyl(2,2-diethoxyvinyl)stannane (entry 5). This issue was successfully overcome by switching from CuI to copper(I) thiophene-2-carboxylate (CuTC), and **19** was obtained with 60% yield and with good reproducibility (entry 6) [87].

Based upon the Stille coupling strategy, Du Bois and co-workers achieved a total synthesis of SEA (**9**), as shown in Scheme 2, including the synthesis of vinyl halide **17** as a substrate for the Stille coupling reaction. Firstly, vinyl halide **17** was synthesized from **20** via Mislow–Evans [2,3] rearrangement: bisguanidine **20** was converted to *N,S*-acetal **21** by reaction with benzenethiol in the presence of BF$_3$·Et$_2$O with 84% yield. Upon treatment of **21** with urea–hydrogen peroxide (UHP), the Mislow–Evans [2,3] rearrangement reaction [88,89] took place under heating in the presence of sodium benzenthiolate, and allylic alcohol **23** was obtained with 81% yield in two steps. After oxidation of the alcohol with Dess–Martin periodinate, the resulting enone **24** was reacted with iodine in the presence of pyridine to give vinyl iodide **17** [90,91], which was further elaborated to **19** by Stille coupling reaction with **25** with 60% yield. Then, the double bond in enone **19** was hydrogenated under high pressure in the presence of Crabtree catalyst **26**. Deprotection of the *tert*-butyldiphenylchlorosilane (TBDPS) ether in **27** with tetrabutylammonium (TBAF) was followed by installation of a carbamoyl group on the resulting hydroxyl group. Finally, deprotection of Tces and Troc and hydrolysis of the ester group were carried out to give (+)-SEA (**9**).

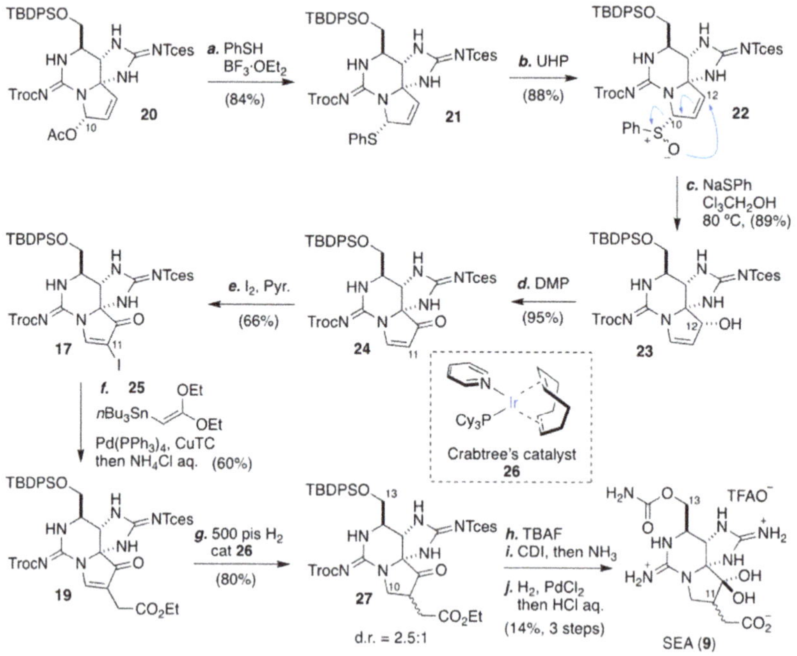

Scheme 2. Introduction of substituent at C11 by Stille coupling, leading to total synthesis of (+)-SEA (**9**) by Du Bois' group.

Table 3. Stille-based cross-coupling conditions with iodoenaminone **17**.

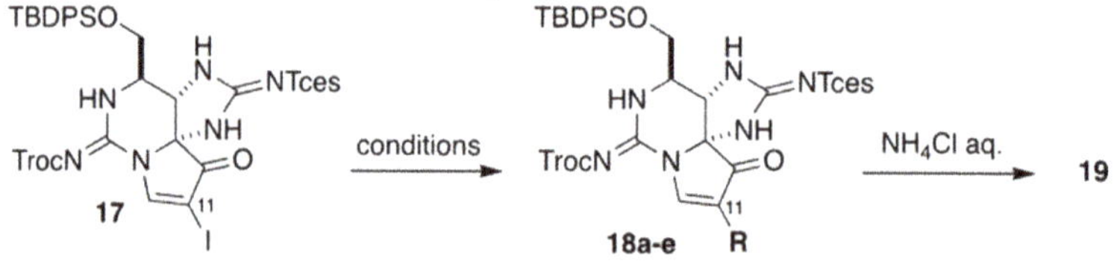

Entry	Conditions	R	Result
1	CH$_2$C(OZnBr)OtBu, Pd$_2$(dba)$_3$/dppf, THF	CH$_2$CO$_2$tBu	**18a** (decomp.)
2	CH$_2$C(OSnnBu$_3$)OEt, PdCl$_2$(P(o-tol)$_3$)$_2$, CuF$_2$	CH$_2$CO$_2$Et	**18b** (N.R.)
3	nBu$_3$SnCH=CH$_2$, Pd(PPh$_3$)$_4$, CuI	CH=CH$_2$	**18c** (< 5%)
4	nBu$_3$SnCH=CH(OEt), Pd(PPh$_3$)$_4$, CuCl, LiCl, THF	CH=CH(OEt)	**18d** (67%)
5	nBu$_3$SnCH=C(OEt)$_2$, Pd(PPh$_3$)$_4$, CuCl, LiCl, THF	CH=C(OEt)$_2$	**19** (0–40%)
6	nBu$_3$SnCH=C(OEt)$_2$, Pd(PPh$_3$)$_4$, CuTC, THF	CH=C(OEt)$_2$	**19** (60%)

CuTC = Copper (I) thiophene-2-carboxylate.

2.3. Carbon–Carbon Bond Formation at C11 by C-Alkylation, As Applied for The Synthesis of (+)-SEA by Looper's Group

In 2019, Looper and co-workers successfully constructed a carbon–carbon bond at C11 in STX, and reported a total synthesis of SEA (**9**) [69]. They initially examined C-alkylation with ketone **28** and electrophiles in the presence of variety of bases, such as lithium bis(trimethylsilyl)amide (LHMDS), lithium diisopropyl amide (LDA), potassium bis(trimethylsilyl)amide (KHMDS) and sodium bis(trimethylsilyl)amide (NaHMDS). In addition, they examined various electrophiles (haloacetates, allylic halides, and propargylic halides), but no reaction took place, as Nagasawa and co-workers had found (Scheme 3) [67].

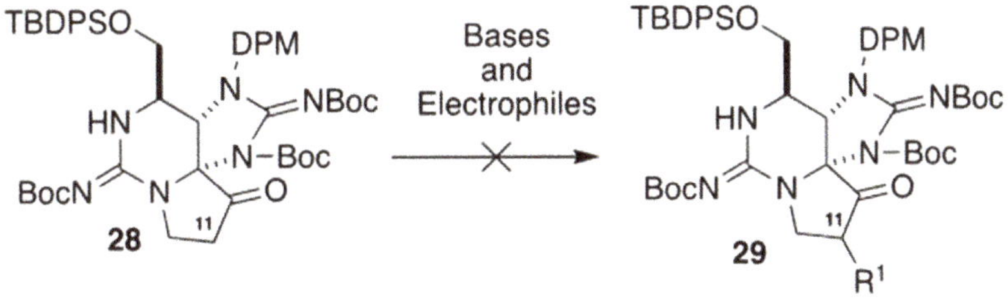

Scheme 3. Examination of carbon–carbon bond construction at C11 by alkylation with ketone **28** in the presence of bases.

On the other hand, they found that C-alkylation took place upon reaction of ketone **28** and *tert*-butyl bromoacetate via the generation of zinc enolate by reaction with LiHMDS in the presence of Et$_2$Zn, affording a mixture of **29a** and its Boc-deprotected derivative **29b** with 60% yield (based on the starting material) (Scheme 4). By means of this alkylation strategy, they succeeded in synthesizing ZTX (**9**) as follows. Deprotection of TBDPS ether in **29** with TBAF followed by carbamoylation of the resulting alcohol resulted in **30**. Finally, total synthesis of SEA (**9**) was achieved by reaction with TFA to hydrolyze the ester and deprotect the Boc and DPM groups.

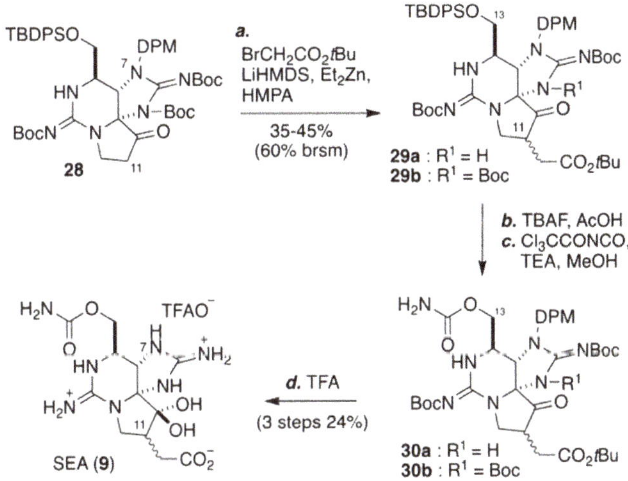

Scheme 4. Carbon–carbon bond formation at C11 by C-alkylation, and total synthesis of (+)-SEA (**9**) by Looper's group.

2.4. Na$_V$-Inhibitory Activity of Synthesized, C11-Substituted Saxitoxin Analogs

Based on the method described above for constructing a carbon–carbon bond at C11 in STX, Nagasawa and co-workers synthesized a series of STX analogs bearing substituents at C11, and evaluated the Na$_V$-inhibitory activity of these analogs at the cellular level [67].

Beside SEA (**9**), they synthesized dicarbamoyl SEA (dcSEA, **31**), 11-saxitoxin ethyl ethanoate (SEE, **32**), and 11-benzylidene STX (**33a**), and evaluated their Na$_V$-inhibitory activity in mouse neuroblastoma Neuro 2A cells, which is known to express Na$_V$1.2, 1.3, 1.4, and 1.7 [70]. SEA (**9**) showed potent inhibitory activity with an IC$_{50}$ value of 47 ± 12 nM, which is twice as potent as decarbamoyl saxitoxin (dcSTX (**3**), IC$_{50}$ = 89 ± 36 M) (Figure 7, Table 4). The dcSEA (**31**) and SEE (**32**) showed IC$_{50}$ values of 5700 ± 3.1 and 185 ± 74 nM, respectively. Interestingly, 11-benzylidene STX (**33a**) was a potent inhibitor, with an IC$_{50}$ value of 16.0 ± 6.9 nM. Although the inhibition mode of **33a** has not been clarified yet, the non-hydrated keto group at C12 in **33** might bind efficiently with Na$_V$, resulting in potent inhibitory activity.

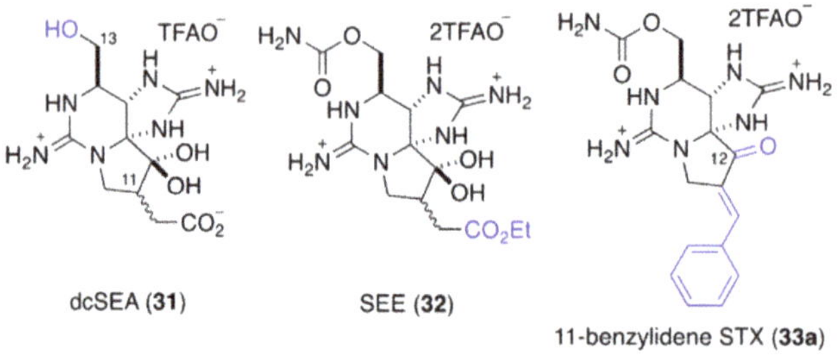

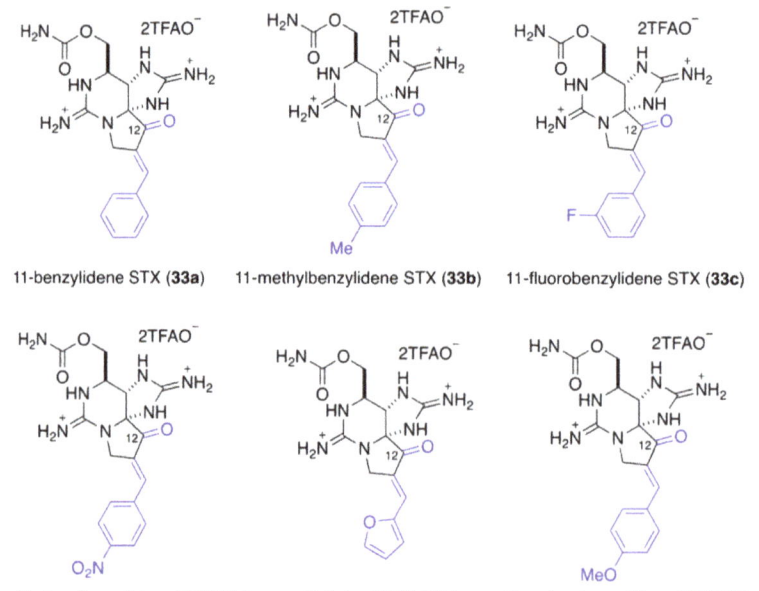

Figure 7. Structures of 9, 31, 32, and 33a.

Table 4. Na$_V$-inhibitory activity of **9**, **31**, **32**, and **33a** in a cell-based assay with Neuro 2A cells.

Compound	IC$_{50}$ (mean ± SD) (nM)	n
dcSTX (**3**)	89 ± 36	3
SEA (**9**)	47 ± 12	3
dcSEA (**31**)	5700 ± 3.1	3
SEE (**32**)	185 ± 74	4
11-benzylidene STX (**33a**)	16 ± 6.9	5

Next, they further synthesized 11-substituted STX analogs **33b–f**, and elucidated their subtype selectivity towards Na$_V$1.2, 1.5, and 1.7, using the whole-cell patch-clamp recording method (Figure 8, Table 5) [92]. They found that 11-fluorobenzylidene STX (**33c**) showed selective and potent inhibitory activity against Na$_V$1.2 (IC$_{50}$ = 7.7 ± 1.6 nM), compared to the other subtypes tested. 11-Benzylidene STX (**33a**) and 11- nitrobenzylidene STX (**33d**) showed potent inhibitory activity against Na$_V$1.5, with IC$_{50}$ values of 94.1 ± 12.0 nM and 50.9 ± 7.8 nM, respectively. These compounds are the most potent TTX-r modulators among STX derivatives so far reported, except for ZTX (**8**) [49].

Figure 8. Structures of 33a–f.

Table 5. Na$_V$-inhibitory activities of **33a–f**, using whole-cell, patch-clamp recording.

Compound	hNa$_V$1.2	hNa$_V$1.5	hNa$_V$1.7
11-benzylidene STX (**33a**)	5.2 ± 6.0	94.1 ± 12.0	124.1 ± 20.6
11-methylbenzylidene STX (**33b**)	22.9 ± 8.6	>300	>300
11-fluorobenzylidene STX (**33c**)	7.7 ± 1.6	>300	>300
11-nitrobenzylidene STX (**33d**)	8.79 ± 0.96	50.9 ± 7.8	>300
11-furfuryl STX (**33e**)	542.7 ± 65.7	>300	>300
11-metoxybenzylidene STX (**33f**)	45.0 ±2.72	>300	>300

IC$_{50}$ (mean ± SD) (nM).

3. Stereoselective Synthesis of The Isoxazolidine Moiety of ZTX (8), And Its Introduction at C13 in A Model Compound

As described in the introduction, ZTX (**8**) has a characteristic macrolactam structure from C6 to C11, involving an isoxazolidine ring system. Thus, stereoselective synthesis of the di-substituted isoxazolidine unit in ZTX (**8**) has been examined. In the paper reporting the isolation of **8** in 2004, the amide carbonyl group in ZTX (**8**) at C13 appeared at 156.5 ppm in the ^{13}C nuclear magnetic resonance (NMR) spectrum, which is a higher chemical shift compared to other amide carbonyls [49]. This interesting observation might be attributed to the unusual macrolactam structure in ZTX (**8**), and synthetic studies of model compounds have been carried out to understand the origin of this unusual chemical shift. In the following section, we discuss the stereoselective isoxazolidine syntheses reported by Nishikawa's [93] and Lopper's groups [94].

3.1. Synthesis of The Isoxazolidine Part of Zetekitoxin (8) from D-ribose by Nishikawa And Co-workers

In 2009, Nishikawa and co-workers reported the stereoselective synthesis of isoxazolidine **42** from D-ribose (**34**) (Scheme 5) [93]. They firstly synthesized nitroolefin **36** from aldehyde **35**, which was derived from D-ribose (**34**) by means of a Henry reaction followed by dehydration with mesylation. After reduction of the double bond in **36** with NaBH$_4$, the resulting nitroalkane **37** was treated with Boc$_2$O to produce dihydrooxazole **39a** and **39b** with 86% yield, as a diastereomeric mixture at C16 in a ratio of 3:1. In this reaction, nitrile oxide **38** was generated first, and a 1,3-dipolar cyclization reaction occurred simultaneously. The major transition state model is shown in Scheme 5. The major diastereomer **39a** was reduced stereoselectively with NaBH$_3$CN to isoxazolidine **40**. After acetylation of the amine in **40**, isoxazolidine **42**, which has the same stereochemistry as ZTX at C15 and C16, was obtained in three steps: (1) deprotection of acetonide with TFA, (2) oxidative cleavage of diol with NaIO$_4$, and (3) reduction of the resulting aldehyde with NaBH$_4$.

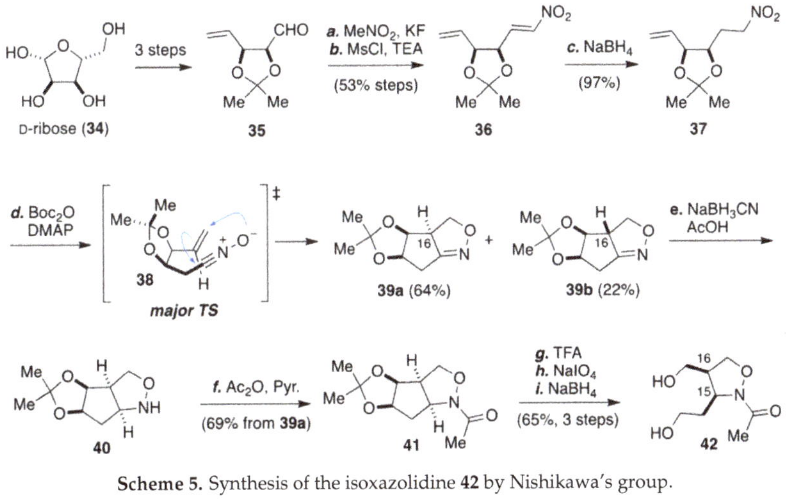

Scheme 5. Synthesis of the isoxazolidine **42** by Nishikawa's group.

3.2. Stereoselective Synthesis of The Isoxazolidine Part from Methyl α-ᴅ-glucopyranoside by Lopper and Co-Workers

In 2015, Lopper and co-workers reported a synthesis of isoxazolidine **59** (Scheme 6) [94]. Aldehyde **45** was synthesized from commercially available methyl α-ᴅ-glucopyranoside (**43**) by the iodination of **44** with iodine and PPh₃, acetylation of the hydroxyl group, and reductive cleavage of the pyran ring with zinc in acetic acid [95]. Then, intramolecular 1,3-dipolar reaction of the terminal olefin with nitrone, which was generated from aldehyde **45** by reaction with hydroxylamine **46**, took place stereoselectively to afford **48** via **47** with 52% yield. After deprotection of acetate in **48** with sodium methoxide [96,97], the resulting triol **49** was treated with NaOI₄ followed by LiAlH₄ to give diol **51** with 70% yield in two steps [98,99]. The isoxazolidine synthon **59** in ZTX (**8**) was synthesized from diol **51** in seven steps by selective functionalization of the two hydroxyl groups, followed by N-acylation.

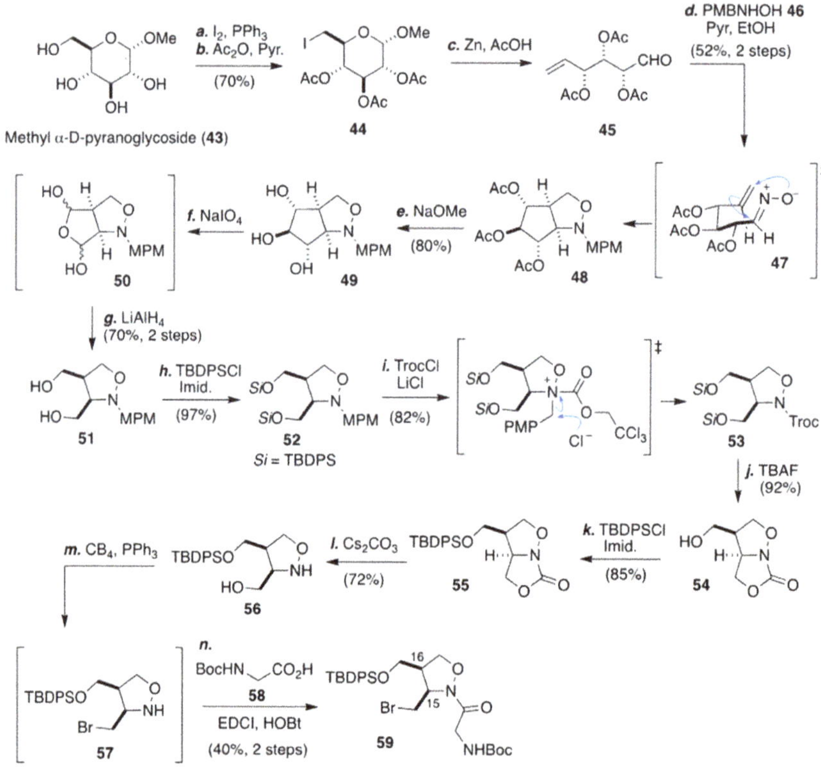

Scheme 6. Synthesis of N-acyl isoxazolidine **59** by Looper's group.

3.3. Comparison of the Chemical Shift at C13 in Zetekitoxin (8) with Those in Some Synthetic Models

As discussed above, the ¹³C NMR chemical shift of the carbonyl group at C13 in ZTX (**8**) has been observed at 156.5 ppm [49], which is a higher value compared with usual amide carbonyl groups (170–175 ppm). To address the issue, Nishikawa's and Looper's groups independently examined the ¹³C chemical shifts of the carbonyl group at C13 in some model compounds (Figure 9) [93,94]. Simple N-acyl isoxazolidine models **60**, **42**, and **59** showed chemical shifts of 171.0, 172.7, 171.0 ppm, respectively, which are quite similar to those of regular cyclic N-acyl amides. However, model compounds **61–63** bearing alpha-guanidinoacetyl amide groups showed chemical shifts of 166.0, 168.3, and 167.0 ppm, respectively, being shifted ca. 5 ppm upfield compared to the other simple models.

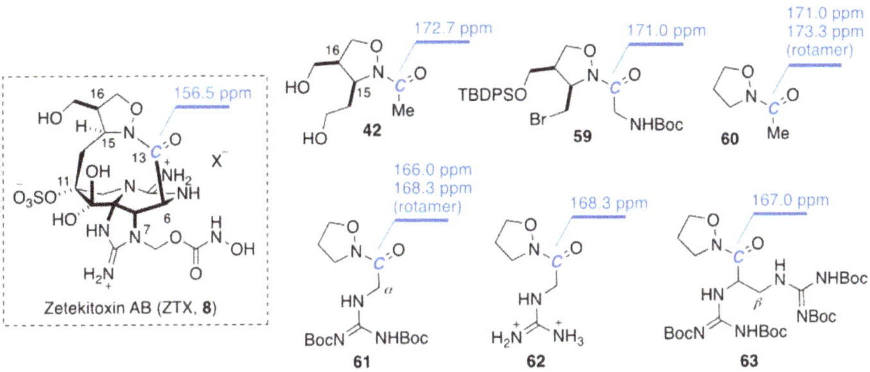

Figure 9. ^{13}C-NMR chemical shifts of ZTX (**8**) and model compounds.

Nagasawa and co-workers examined the chemical shift at C13 of **70**, which has an STX skeleton; its synthesis is depicted in Scheme 7 [100]. They firstly aimed to obtain carboxylic acid **66** from alcohol **64** by oxidation. They examined various oxidants and conditions, but it appeared that the hydroxyl group in **64** was unreactive due to its axial orientation, and no reaction occurred, or unexpected side reactions proceeded. Finally, they found that 2-azaadamantane N-oxyl (AZADO)–NaClO and NaClO$_2$ [101,102] were effective, resulting in carboxylic acid **66**, which was obtained with 79% yield after TMSCHN$_2$ treatment of the crude carboxylic acid **66** to hydrolyze the methyl ester **67**. Condensation of carboxylic acid **66** with isoxazolidine **40** [93] in the presence of 4-(4, 6- dimethoxy-1,3,5-triazin-2-yl)-4-methylmorpholinium chloride (DMT-MM,**68**) [103], followed by deprotection of the Boc group and acetal with TFA, gave amide **70** in 98% yield. Unfortunately, the chemical shift of the carbonyl group in **70** was observed at 166.1 ppm, slightly higher than that of **62** or **63**, but still lower than that of ZTX (**8**). The chemical shift in ZTX (**8**) may reflect the characteristic spatial structure associated with the presence of the macrolactam moiety.

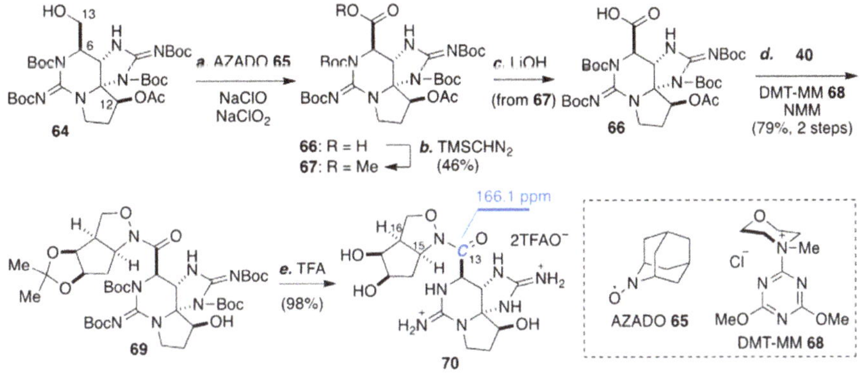

Scheme 7. Oxidation at C13 and introduction of the isoxazolidine motif.

4. Synthesis of The Characteristic Macrocyclic Structure of ZTX (8) by Looper's Group

Looper and co-workers have reported macrocyclic compound **72** as a model for ZTX (**8**) (Scheme 8) [71]. After deprotection of the TBDPS ether group at C13 with TBAF, the resulting alcohol was reacted with iodoacetic acid in the presence of 1-(3-dimethylaminopropyl)-3-ethylcarbodiimide (EDC) and N,N-dimethyl-4-aminopyridine (DMAP) to give iodoester **71** with 58% yield. When iodoester **71** was treated with a strong base, *tert*-butylimino-tri(pyrrolidino)phosphorane (BTPP), intramolecular alkylation proceeded at C11, and the corresponding macrolactone **72** was obtained in 48% yield. It should be possible to construct the macrolactam structure of **8** via a similar strategy, and this should also resolve the chemical shift issue in ZTX (**8**).

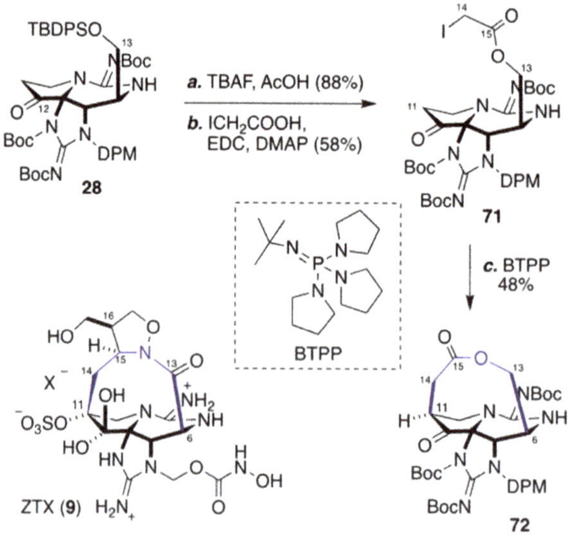

Scheme 8. Synthesis of macrolactone **72** via intramolecular alkylation by Looper's group.

5. Conclusions

Here, we have reviewed recent progress towards the total synthesis of zetekitoxin AB (**8**, ZTX). Although this goal still remains elusive, there have been some significant synthetic advances in the construction of characteristic structures of ZTX, such as (i) the carbon–carbon bond at C11 in the STX structure, (ii) stereoselective construction of the substituted isoxazolidine moiety at C15 and C16, and (iii) the macrocyclic structure from C6 to C11. Since ZTX has potent inhibitory activity, even towards tetrodotoxin-resistant (TTX-r) Na$_V$s, a total synthesis of ZTX and its analogs is expected to provide useful tools for chemical biological studies of Na$_V$s, overcoming the severely restricted availability of natural ZTX.

Author Contributions: Conceived and designed the story of manuscript, K.N.; writing–original draft preparation, K.N. and M.O.; writing—review and editing, K.A., H.I., M.O. All authors have read and agreed to the published version of the manuscript.

Funding: This research was funded by Grants-in-Aid for Scientific Research on Innovative Areas "Middle Molecular Strategy" (18H04387 to K.N.), Grants-in-Aid for Scientific Research (B) (JP26282214 to K.N.), and the A3-foresight program. M.O. thanks the Japan Society for the Promotion of Science (JSPS), KAKENHI Grant Number 18K14210. This work was inspired by the international and interdisciplinary environment of the JSPS Asian CORE Program of ACBI (Asian Chemical Biology Initiative).

Acknowledgments: K.A. thanks SUNBOR for providing a scholarship.

Conflicts of Interest: The authors declare no conflict of interest.

References

1. Hodgkin, A.L.; Huxley, A.F. A quantitative description of membrane current and its application to conduction and excitation in nerve. *J. Physiol.* **1952**, *117*, 500–544. [CrossRef] [PubMed]
2. Goldin, A.L.; Barchi, R.L.; Caldwell, J.H.; Hofmann, F.; Howe, J.R.; Hunter, J.C.; Kallen, R.G.; Mandel, G.; Meisler, M.H.; Netter, Y.B.; et al. Nomenclature of voltage-gated sodium channels. *Neuron* **2000**, *28*, 365–368. [CrossRef]
3. Narahashi, T. Tetrodotoxin. *Proc. Jpn. Acad. Ser. B* **2008**, *84*, 147–154. [CrossRef] [PubMed]

4. Nishikawa, T.; Isobe, M. Synthesis of Tetrodotoxin, a Classic but Still Fascinating Natural Product. *Chem. Rec.* **2013**, *13*, 286–302. [CrossRef]

5. Moczydlowski, E.G. The molecular mystique of tetrodotoxin. *Toxicon* **2013**, *63*, 165–183. [CrossRef]

6. Fozzard, H.A.; Lipkind, G.M. The Tetrodotoxin Binding Site Is within the Outer Vestibule of the Sodium Channel. *Mar. Drugs* **2010**, *8*, 219–234. [CrossRef]

7. Lee, C.H.; Ruben, P.C. Interaction between voltage-gated sodium channels and the neurotoxin, tetrodotoxin. *Channels* **2008**, *2*, 407–412. [CrossRef]

8. Clare, J.J.; Tate, S.N.; Nobbs, M.; Romanos, M.A. Voltage-gated sodium channels as therapeutic targets. *Drug Discov. Today* **2000**, *5*, 506–520. [CrossRef]

9. Noda, M.; Ikeda, T.; Kayano, T.; Suzuki, H.; Takeshima, H.; Kurasaki, M.; Takahashi, H.; Numa, S. Existence of distinct sodium channel messenger RNAs in rat brain. *Nature* **1986**, *320*, 188–192. [CrossRef]

10. Meadows, L.S.; Chen, Y.H.; Powell, A.J.; Clare, J.J.; Ragsdale, D.S. Functional modulation of human brain $Na_V1.3$ sodium channels, expressed in mammalian cells, by auxiliary beta 1, beta 2 and beta 3 subunits. *Neuroscience* **2002**, *114*, 745–753. [CrossRef]

11. Trimmer, J.S.; Cooperman, S.S.; Tomiko, S.A.; Zhou, J.; Crean, S.M.; Boyle, M.B.; Kallen, R.G.; Sheng, Z.; Barchi, R.L.; Sigworth, F.J. Primary structure and functional expression of a mammalian skeletal muscle sodium channel. *Neuron* **1989**, *3*, 33–49. [CrossRef]

12. Chahine, M.; Bennett, P.B.; George, A.L., Jr.; Horn, R. Functional expression and properties of the human skeletal muscle sodium channel. *Pflug. Arch. Eur. J. Physiol.* **1994**, *427*, 136–142. [CrossRef] [PubMed]

13. Dietrich, P.S.; McGivern, J.G.; Delgado, S.G.; Koch, B.D.; Eglen, R.M.; Hunter, J.C.; Sangameswaran, L. Functional analysis of a voltage-gated sodium channel and its splice variant from rat dorsal root ganglia. *J. Neurochem.* **1998**, *70*, 2262–2272. [CrossRef] [PubMed]

14. Smith, M.R.; Smith, R.D.; Plummer, N.W.; Meisler, M.H.; Goldin, A.L. Functional Analysis of the Mouse Scn8a Sodium Channel. *J. Neurosci.* **1998**, *18*, 6093–6102. [CrossRef] [PubMed]

15. Klugbauer, N.; Lacinova, L.; Flockerzi, V.; Hofmann, F. Structure and functional expression of a new member of the tetrodotoxin-sensitive voltage-activated sodium channel family from human neuroendocrine cells. *EMBO J.* **1995**, *14*, 1084–1090. [CrossRef] [PubMed]

16. Cummins, T.R.; Howe, J.R.; Waxman, S.G. Slow Closed-State Inactivation: A Novel Mechanism Underlying Ramp Currents in Cells Expressing the hNE/PN1 Sodium Channel. *J. Neurosci.* **1998**, *18*, 9607–9619. [CrossRef]

17. Sangameswaran, L.; Fish, L.M.; Koch, B.D.; Rabert, D.K.; Delgado, S.G.; Ilnicka, M.; Jakeman, L.B.; Novakovic, S.; Wong, K.; Sze, P.; et al. A Novel Tetrodotoxin-sensitive, Voltage-gated Sodium Channel Expressed in Rat and Human Dorsal Root Ganglia. *J. Biol. Chem.* **1997**, *272*, 14805–14809. [CrossRef]

18. Santarelli, V.P.; Eastwood, A.L.; Dougherty, D.A.; Horn, R.; Ahern, C.A. A cation-pi interaction discriminates among sodium channels that are either sensitive or resistant to tetrodotoxin block. *J. Biol. Chem.* **2007**, *282*, 8044–8051. [CrossRef]

19. Satin, J.; Kyle, J.W.; Chen, M.; Bell, P.; Cribbs, L.L.; Fozzard, H.A.; Rogart, R.B. A Mutant of TTX-Resistant Cardiac Sodium Channels with TTX-Sensitive Properties. *Science* **1992**, *256*, 1202–1205. [CrossRef]

20. Sangameswaran, L.; Delgado, S.G.; Fish, L.M.; Koch, B.D.; Jakeman, L.B.; Stewart, G.R.; Sze, P.; Hunter, J.C.; Eglen, R.M.; Herman, R.C. Structure and Function of a Novel Voltage-gated, Tetrodotoxin-resistant Sodium Channel Specific to Sensory Neurons. *J. Biol. Chem.* **1996**, *271*, 5953–5956. [CrossRef]

21. Akopian, A.N.; Sivilotti, L.; Wood, J.N. A tetrodotoxin-resistant voltage-gated sodium channel expressed by sensory neurons. *Nature* **1996**, *379*, 257–262. [CrossRef] [PubMed]

22. Dib-Hajj, S.D.; Tyrrell, L.; Black, J.A.; Waxman, S.G. NaN, a novel voltage-gated Na channel, is expressed preferentially in peripheral sensory neurons and down-regulated after axotomy. *Proc. Natl. Acad. Sci. USA* **1998**, *95*, 8963–8968. [CrossRef] [PubMed]

23. Dib-Hajj, S.; Black, J.A.; Cummins, T.R.; Waxman, S.G. NaN/$Na_V1.9$: A sodium channel with unique properties. *Trends Neurosci.* **2002**, *25*, 253–259. [CrossRef]

24. McKerrall, S.J.; Sutherlin, D.P. $Na_V1.7$ inhibitors for the treatment of chronic pain. *Bioorg. Med. Chem. Lett.* **2018**, *28*, 3141–3149. [CrossRef] [PubMed]

25. Mulcahy, J.V.; Pajouhesh, H.; Beckley, J.T.; Delwig, A.; Du Bois, J.; Hunter, J.C. Challenges and Opportunities for Therapeutics Targeting the Voltage-Gated Sodium Channel Isoform $Na_V1.7$. *J. Med. Chem.* **2019**, *62*, 8695–8710. [CrossRef] [PubMed]

26. Bagal, S.K.; Kemp, M.L.; Bungay, P.J.; Hay, T.L.; Murata, Y.; Payne, C.E.; Stevens, E.B.; Brown, A.; Blakemore, D.C.; Corbett, M.S.; et al. Discovery and optimisation of potent and highly subtype selective Na$_V$1.8 inhibitors with reduced cardiovascular liabilities. *Med. Chem. Comm.* **2016**, *7*, 1925–1931. [CrossRef]

27. Kort, M.E.; Atkinson, R.N.; Thomas, J.B.; Drizin, I.; Johnson, M.S.; Secrest, M.A.; Gregg, R.J.; Scanio, M.J.; Shi, L.; Hakeem, A.H.; et al. Subtype-selective Na$_V$1.8 sodium channel blockers: Identification of potent, orally active nicotinamide derivatives. *Bioorg. Med. Chem. Let.* **2010**, *20*, 6812–6815. [CrossRef]

28. Jarvis, M.F.; Honore, P.; Shieh, C.C.; Chapman, M.; Joshi, S.; Zhang, X.F.; Kort, M.; Carroll, W.; Marron, B.; Atkinson, R.; et al. A-803467, a potent and selective Na$_V$1.8 sodium channel blocker, attenuates neuropathic and inflammatory pain in the rat. *Proc. Natl. Acad. Sci. USA* **2007**, *104*, 8520–8525. [CrossRef]

29. Kort, M.E.; Drizin, I.; Gregg, R.J.; Scanio, M.J.; Shi, L.; Gross, M.F.; Atkinson, R.N.; Johnson, M.S.; Pacofsky, G.J.; Thomas, J.B.; et al. Discovery and biological evaluation of 5-aryl-2-furfuramides, potent and selective blockers of the Na$_V$1.8 sodium channel with efficacy in models of neuropathic and inflammatory pain. *J. Med. Chem.* **2008**, *51*, 407–416. [CrossRef]

30. Priest, B.T.; Kaczorowski, G.J. Subtype-selective sodium channel blockers promise a new era of pain research. *Proc. Natl. Acad. Sci. USA* **2007**, *104*, 8205–8206. [CrossRef]

31. England, S.; de Groot, M.J. Subtype-selective targeting of voltage-gated sodium channels. *Br. J. Pharm.* **2009**, *158*, 1413–1425. [CrossRef] [PubMed]

32. Llewellyn, L.E. Saxitoxin, a toxic marine natural product that targets a multitude of receptors. *Nat. Prod. Rep.* **2006**, *23*, 200–222. [CrossRef] [PubMed]

33. Cusick, K.D.; Sayler, G.S. An Overview on the Marine Neurotoxin, Saxitoxin: Genetics, Molecular Targets, Methods of Detection and Ecological Functions. *Mar. Drugs* **2013**, *11*, 991–1018. [CrossRef] [PubMed]

34. Sommer, H.; Meyer, G.F. Paralytic shellfish poisoning. *Arch. Pathol.* **1937**, *24*, 560–598.

35. Sommer, H.; Whedon, W.F.; Kofoid, C.A.; Strohler, R. Relation of paralytic shellfish poison to certain plankton organisms of the genus Gonyaulax. *Arch. Pathol.* **1937**, *24*, 537–559.

36. Schantz, E.J.; Mold, J.D.; Stanger, D.W.; Shavel, J.; Riel, F.J.; Bowden, J.P.; Lynch, J.M.; Wyler, R.S.; Riegel, B.; Sommer, H. Paralytic Shellfish Poison. VI. A Procedure for the Isolation and Purification of the Poison from Toxic Clam and Mussel Tissues. *J. Am. Chem. Soc.* **1957**, *79*, 5230–5235. [CrossRef]

37. Mold, J.D.; Bowden, J.P.; Stanger, D.W.; Maurer, J.E.; Lynch, J.M.; Wyler, R.S.; Schantz, E.J.; Riegel, B. Paralytic Shellfish Poison. VII. Evidence for the Purity of the Poison Isolated from Toxic Clams and Mussels. *J. Am. Chem. Soc.* **1957**, *79*, 5235–5238. [CrossRef]

38. Schuett, W.; Rapoport, H. Saxitoxin, the Paralytic Shellfish Poison. Degradation to a Pyrrolopyrimidine. *J. Am. Chem. Soc.* **1962**, *84*, 2266–2267. [CrossRef]

39. Russell, F.E. Comparative pharmacology of some animal toxins. *Fed. Proc.* **1967**, *26*, 1206–1224.

40. Bordner, J.; Thiessen, W.E.; Bates, H.A.; Rapoport, H. Structure of a crystalline derivative of saxitoxin. Structure of saxitoxin. *J. Am. Chem. Soc.* **1975**, *97*, 6008–6012. [CrossRef]

41. Rogers, P.S.; Rapoport, H. The pKa's of saxitoxin. *J. Am. Chem. Soc.* **1980**, *102*, 7335–7339. [CrossRef]

42. Henderson, R.; Ritchie, J.M.; Strichartz, G.R. Evidence that tetrodotoxin and saxitoxin act at a metal cation binding site in the sodium channels of nerve membrane. *Proc. Natl. Acad. Sci. USA* **1974**, *71*, 3936–3940. [CrossRef] [PubMed]

43. Hille, B. The receptor for tetrodotoxin and saxitoxin. A structural hypothesis. *Biophys. J.* **1975**, *15*, 615–619. [PubMed]

44. Pan, X.; Li, Z.; Zhou, Q.; Shen, H.; Wu, K.; Huang, X.; Chen, J.; Zhang, J.; Zhu, X.; Lei, J.; et al. Structural basis for the modulation of voltage-gated sodium channels by animal toxins. *Science* **2018**, *362*, eaau2596.

45. Shen, H.; Liu, D.; Wu, K.; Lei, J.; Yan, N. Structures of human Na$_V$1.7 channel in complex with auxiliary subunits and animal toxins. *Science* **2019**, *363*, 1303–1308. [CrossRef] [PubMed]

46. Walker, J.R.; Novick, P.A.; Parsons, W.H.; McGregor, M.; Zablocki, J.; Pande, V.S.; Du Bois, J. Marked difference in saxitoxin and tetrodotoxin affinity for the human nociceptive voltage-gated sodium channel (Na$_V$1.7). *Proc. Natl. Acad. Sci. USA* **2012**, *109*, 18102–18107. [CrossRef]

47. Thomas-Tran, R.; Du Bois, J. Mutant cycle analysis with modified saxitoxins reveals specific interactions critical to attaining high-affinity inhibition of hNa$_V$1.7. *Proc. Natl. Acad. Sci. USA* **2016**, *113*, 5856–5861. [CrossRef]

48. Wiese, M.; D'Agostino, P.M.; Mihali, T.K.; Moffitt, M.C.; Neilan, B.A. Neurotoxic Alkaloids: Saxitoxin and Its Analogs. *Mar. Drugs* **2010**, *8*, 2185–2211. [CrossRef]

49. Yotsu-Yamashita, M.; Kim, Y.H.; Dudley, S.C., Jr.; Choudhary, G.; Pfahnl, A.; Oshima, Y.; Daly, J.W. The structure of zetekitoxin AB, a saxitoxin analog from the Panamanian golden frog Atelopus zeteki: A potent sodium-channel blocker. *Proc. Natl. Acad. Sci. USA* **2004**, *101*, 4346–4351. [CrossRef]

50. Fuhrman, F.A.; Fuhrman, G.J.; Mosher, H.S. Toxin from Skin of Frogs of the Genus Atelopus: Differentiation from Dendrobatid Toxins. *Science* **1969**, *165*, 1376–1377. [CrossRef]

51. Shindelman, J.; Mosher, H.S.; Fuhrman, F.A. Atelopidtoxin from the Panamanian frog, Atelopus Zeteki. *Toxicon* **1969**, *7*, 315–319. [CrossRef]

52. Tanino, H.; Nakada, T.; Kaneko, Y.; Kishi, Y. A stereospecific total synthesis of dl-saxitoxin. *J. Am. Chem. Soc.* **1977**, *99*, 2818–2819. [CrossRef] [PubMed]

53. Jacobi, P.A.; Martineli, M.J.; Polanc, S. Total synthesis of (±)-saxitoxin. *J. Am. Chem. Soc.* **1984**, *106*, 5594–5598. [CrossRef]

54. Fleming, J.J.; Du Bois, J. A Synthesis of (+)-Saxitoxin. *J. Am. Chem. Soc.* **2006**, *128*, 3926–3927. [CrossRef]

55. Iwamoto, O.; Koshino, H.; Hashizume, D.; Nagasawa, K. Total synthesis of (−)-decarbamoyloxysaxitoxin. *Angew. Chem. Int. Ed.* **2007**, *46*, 8625–8628. [CrossRef]

56. Mulcahy, J.V.; Du Bois, J. A Stereoselective Synthesis of (+)-Gonyautoxin 3. *J. Am. Chem. Soc.* **2008**, *130*, 12630–12631. [CrossRef]

57. Iwamoto, O.; Shinohara, R.; Nagasawa, K. Total Synthesis of (−)- and (+)-Decarbamoyloxysaxitoxin and (+)-Saxitoxin. *Chem. Asian J.* **2009**, *4*, 277–285. [CrossRef]

58. Iwamoto, O.; Nagasawa, K. Total Synthesis of (+)-Decarbamoylsaxitoxin and (+)-Gonyautoxin 3. *Org. Lett.* **2010**, *12*, 2150–2153. [CrossRef]

59. Sawayama, Y.; Nishikawa, T. A Synthetic Route to the Saxitoxin Skeleton: Synthesis of Decarbamoyl α-Saxitoxinol, an Analogue of Saxitoxin Produced by the Cyanobacterium Lyngbya wollei. *Angew. Chem. Int. Ed.* **2011**, *50*, 7176–7178. [CrossRef]

60. Bhonde, V.R.; Looper, R.E. A Stereocontrolled Synthesis of (+)-Saxitoxin. *J. Am. Chem. Soc.* **2011**, *133*, 20172–20174. [CrossRef]

61. Mulcahy, J.V.; Walker, J.R.; Merit, J.E.; Whitehead, A.; Du Bois, J. Synthesis of the Paralytic Shellfish Poisons (+)-Gonyautoxin 2, (+)-Gonyautoxin 3, and (+)-11,11-Dihydroxysaxitoxin. *J. Am. Chem. Soc.* **2016**, *138*, 5994–6001. [CrossRef] [PubMed]

62. Thottumkara, A.P.; Parsons, W.H.; Du Bois, J. Saxitoxin. *Angew. Chem. Int. Ed.* **2014**, *53*, 5760–5784. [CrossRef] [PubMed]

63. Andresen, B.M.; Du Bois, J. De Novo Synthesis of Modified Saxitoxins for Sodium Ion Channel Study. *J. Am. Chem. Soc.* **2009**, *131*, 12524–12525. [CrossRef] [PubMed]

64. Parsons, W.H.; Du Bois, J. Maleimide Conjugates of Saxitoxin as Covalent Inhibitors of Voltage-Gated Sodium Channels. *J. Am. Chem. Soc.* **2013**, *135*, 10582–10585. [CrossRef]

65. Akimoto, T.; Masuda, A.; Yotsu-Mari, M.; Hirokawa, T.; Nagasawa, K. Synthesis of saxitoxin derivatives bearing guanidine and urea groups at C13 and evaluation of their inhibitory activity on voltage-gated sodium channels. *Org. Biomol. Chem.* **2013**, *11*, 6642–6649. [CrossRef]

66. Arakawa, O.; Nishio, S.; Noguchi, T.; Shida, Y.; Onoue, Y. A new saxitoxin analogue from a xanthid crab Atergatis Floridus. *Toxicon* **1995**, *12*, 1577–1584. [CrossRef]

67. Wang, C.; Oki, M.; Nishikawa, T.; Harada, D.; Yotsu-Yamashita, M.; Nagasawa, K. Total Synthesis of 11-Saxitoxinethanoic Acid and Evaluation of its Inhibitory Activity on Voltage-gated Sodium Channels. *Angew. Chem. Int. Ed.* **2016**, *55*, 11600–11603. [CrossRef]

68. Walker, R.J.; Merit, E.J.; Thomas-Tran, R.; Tang, D.T.Y.; Du Bois, J. Divergent Synthesis of Natural Derivatives of (+)-Saxitoxin Including 11-Saxitoxinethanoic Acid. *Angew. Chem. Int. Ed.* **2018**, *58*, 1689–1693. [CrossRef]

69. Paladugu, S.R.; James, C.K.; Looper, R.E. A Direct C11 Alkylation Strategy on the Saxitoxin Core: A Synthesis of (+)-11-Saxitoxinethanoic Acid. *Org. Lett.* **2019**, *21*, 7999–8002. [CrossRef]

70. Lou, J.-Y.; Laezza, F.; Gerber, B.R.; Xiao, M.L.; Yamada, K.A.; Hartmann, H.; Craig, A.M.; Nerbonne, J.M.; Ornitz, D.M. Fibroblast growth factor 14 is an intracellular modulator of voltage-gated sodium channels. *J. Physiol.* **2005**, *569*, 179–193. [CrossRef]

71. Matsuo, J.; Murakami, M. The Mukaiyama Aldol Reaction: 40 Years of Continuous Development. *Angew. Chem. Int. Ed.* **2013**, *52*, 9109–9118. [CrossRef] [PubMed]

72. Mase, N.; Hayashi, Y. The Aldol Reaction: Organocatalysis Approach. In *Comprehensive Organic Synthesis*, 2nd ed.; Knochel, P., Molander, G.A., Eds.; Elsevier: Amsterdam, The Netherlands, 2014; Volume 2, pp. 273–339.

73. Hosokawa, S. Recent development of vinylogous Mukaiyama aldol reactions. *Tetrahedron Lett.* **2018**, *59*, 77–88. [CrossRef]

74. Mukaiyama, T.; Narasaka, K.; Banno, K. New aldol type reaction. *Chem. Lett.* **1973**, 1011–1014.

75. Mukaiyama, T.; Banno, K.; Narasaka, K. New cross-aldol reactions. Reactions of silyl enol ethers with carbonyl compounds activated by titanium tetrachloride. *J. Am. Chem. Soc.* **1974**, *96*, 7503–7509. [CrossRef]

76. Noyori, R.; Yokoyama, K.; Sakata, J.; Kuwajima, I.; Nakamura, E.; Shimizu, M. Fluoride ion catalyzed aldol reaction between enol silyl ethers and carbonyl compounds. *J. Am. Chem. Soc.* **1977**, *99*, 1265–1267. [CrossRef]

77. Gingras, M.; Chabre, Y.M.; Raimundo, J.-M. Tetrabutylammonium Difluorotriphenylstannate [Bu$_4$N] [Ph$_3$SnF$_2$]: Delivering Carbon or Fluorine Ligands via Hypercoordination. *Synthesis* **2006**, *1*, 182–185. [CrossRef]

78. Hama, T.; Liu, X.; Culkin, D.A.; Hartwig, J.F. Palladium-Catalyzed α-Arylation of Esters and Amides under More Neutral Conditions. *J. Am. Chem. Soc.* **2003**, *125*, 11176–11177. [CrossRef]

79. Moradi, W.A.; Buchwald, S.L. Palladium-Catalyzed α-Arylation of Esters. *J. Am. Chem. Soc.* **2001**, *123*, 7996–8002. [CrossRef]

80. Magauer, T.; Mulzer, J.; Tiefenbacher, K. Total Syntheses of (+)-Echinopine A and B: Determination of Absolute Stereochemistry. *Org. Lett.* **2009**, *11*, 5306–5309. [CrossRef]

81. Xiao, Q.; Ren, W.-W.; Chen, Z.-X.; Sun, T.-W.; Li, Y.; Ye, Q.-D.; Gong, J.-X.; Meng, F.-K.; You, L.; Liu, Y.-F.; et al. Diastereoselective Total Synthesis of (±)-Schindilactone A. *Angew. Chem. Int. Ed.* **2011**, *50*, 7373–7377. [CrossRef]

82. Negishi, E. Novel and selective α-substitution of ketones and other carbonyl compounds based on Pd-catalyzed cross coupling of α-unsaturated carbonyl derivatives containing α-halogen or α-metal groups. *J. Organomet. Chem.* **1999**, *576*, 179–194. [CrossRef]

83. Johnson, C.R.; Adams, J.P.; Braun, M.P.; Senanayake, C.B.W. Modified stille coupling utilizing α-iodoenones. *Tetrahedron Lett.* **1992**, *33*, 919–922. [CrossRef]

84. Cordvilla, C.; Bartolome, C.; Martinez-Ilarduya, J.M.; Espinet, P. The Stille Reaction, 38 Years Later. *ACS Catal.* **2015**, *5*, 3040–3053. [CrossRef]

85. Han, X.; Stoltz, B.; Corey, E.J. Cuprous Chloride Accelerated Stille Reactions. A General and Effective Coupling System for Sterically Congested Substrates and for Enantioselective Synthesis. *J. Am. Chem. Soc.* **1999**, *121*, 7600–7605. [CrossRef]

86. Devlin, A.S.; Du Bois, J. Modular synthesis of the pentacyclic core of batrachotoxin and select batrachotoxin analogue designs. *Chem. Sci.* **2013**, *4*, 1059–1063. [CrossRef] [PubMed]

87. Allred, G.D.; Liebeskind, L.S. Copper-Mediated Cross-Coupling of Organostannanes with Organic Iodides at or below Room Temperature. *J. Am. Chem. Soc.* **1996**, *118*, 2748–2749. [CrossRef]

88. Colomer, I.; Velado, M.; Fe rnandez de la Pradilla, R.; Viso, A. From Allylic Sulfoxides to Allylic Sulfenates: Fifty Years of a Never-Ending [2,3]-Sigmatropic Rearrangement. *Chem. Rev.* **2017**, *117*, 14201–14243. [CrossRef]

89. Rojas, C.M. The Mislow-Evans rearrangement. In *Molecular Rearrangements in Organic Synthesis*; Rojas, C.M., Ed.; John Wiley & Sons: Hoboken, NJ, USA, 2016. [CrossRef]

90. Johnson, C.R.; Adams, J.P.; Braun, M.P.; Senanayake, C.B.W.; Wovkulich, P.M.; Uskokovic, M.R. Direct α-iodination of cycloalkenones. *Tetrahedron Lett.* **1992**, *33*, 917–918. [CrossRef]

91. Djuardi, E.; Bovonsombat, P.; McNelis, E. Formations of α-Iodoenones by Iodine and Catalytic Amounts of Amines. *Synth. Commun.* **1997**, *27*, 2497–2503. [CrossRef]

92. Adachi, K.; Yamada, T.; Ishizuka, H.; Oki, M.; Tsunogae, S.; Shimada, N.; Chiba, O.; Orihara, T.; Hidaka, M.; Hirokawa, T.; et al. Synthesis of C12-keto saxitoxin derivatives with unusual inhibitory activity against voltage-gated sodium channels. *Chem. Eur. J.* **2019**. [CrossRef]

93. Nishikawa, T.; Urabe, D.; Isobe, M. Syntheses of *N*-Acylisoxazolidine Derivatives, Related to a Partial Structure Found in Zetekitoxin AB, a Golden Frog Poison. *Heterocycles* **2009**, *79*, 379–385. [CrossRef]

94. Paladugu, S.R.; Looper, R.E. Preparation of a 1,2-isoxazolidine synthon for the synthesis of zetekitoxin AB. *Tetrahedron Lett.* **2015**, *56*, 6332–6334. [CrossRef] [PubMed]

95. Bernet, B.; Vasella, A. Carbocyclische Verbindungen aus Monosacchariden. II. Umsetzungen in der Mannosereihe. *Helv. Chim. Acta* **1979**, *62*, 2400–2410. [CrossRef]

96. Ferrier, R.J.; Furneaux, R.H.; Prasit, P.; Tyler, P.C. Functionalised carbocycles from carbohydrates. Part 2. The synthesis of 3-oxa-2-azabicyclo[3.3.0]octanes. X-Ray crystal structure of (1*R*,5*S*)-6-*exo*,7-*endo*,8-*exo*-triacetoxy-*N*-methyl-4-*endo*-phenylthio-3-oxa-2-azabicyclo[3.3.0]octane. *J. Chem. Soc. Perkin Trans. 1* **1983**, *1*, 1621–1628. [CrossRef]

97. Dransfield, P.J.; Moutel, S.; Shipman, M.; Sik, V. Stereocontrolled synthesis of polyhydroxylated hexahydro-1*H*-cyclopent[*c*]isoxazoles by intramolecular oxime olefin cycloadditions: An approach to aminocyclopentitols. *J. Chem. Soc. Perkin Trans. 1* **1999**, *1*, 3349–3355. [CrossRef]

98. Ogawa, S.; Orihara, M. Synthesis of the penta-*N*,*O*-acetyl derivatives of some pseudo-3-amino-3-deoxy-DL-hexopyranoses a and -DL-hexopyranosylamine derivative. *Carbohydr. Res.* **1989**, *189*, 323–330. [CrossRef]

99. Baumgartner, H.; O'Sullivan, A.C.; Schneider, J. The Synthesis of Oxa-Analogs of the Kainoid Family. *Heterocycles* **1997**, *45*, 1537–1549.

100. Nishikawa, T.; Wang, C.; Akimoto, T.; Koshino, H.; Nagasawa, K. Synthesis of an advance model of zetekitoxin AB focusing on *N*-acylisoxazolidine amide structure corresponding to C13–C17. *Asian J. Org. Chem.* **2014**, *3*, 1308–1311. [CrossRef]

101. Shibuya, M.; Tomizawa, M.; Suzuki, I.; Iwabuchi, Y. 2-Azaadamantane *N*-Oxyl (AZADO) and 1-Me-AZADO: Highly Efficient Organocatalysts for Oxidation of Alcohols. *J. Am. Chem. Soc.* **2006**, *128*, 8412–8413. [CrossRef]

102. Shibuya, M.; Sato, T.; Tomizawa, M.; Iwabuchi, Y. Oxoammonium salt/NaClO$_2$: An expedient, catalytic system for one-pot oxidation of primary alcohols to carboxylic acids with broad substrate applicability. *Chem. Commun.* **2009**, *13*, 1739–1741. [CrossRef]

103. Kunishima, M.; Kawachi, C.; Hioki, K.; Tani, S. Formation of carboxamides by direct condensation of carboxylic acids and amines in *alcohols* using a new alcohol- and water-soluble condensing agent: DMT-MM. *Tetrahedron* **2001**, *57*, 1551–1558. [CrossRef]

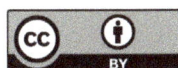

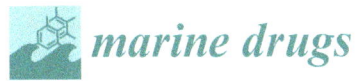

Review

Marine Natural Products and Drug Resistance in Latent Tuberculosis

Muhammad Tahir Khan [1], Aman Chandra Kaushik [2], Aamer Iqbal Bhatti [3], Yu-Juan Zhang [4], Shulin Zhang [5], Amie Jinghua Wei [5], Shaukat Iqbal Malik [1] and Dong Qing Wei [2,*

[1] Department of Bioinformatics and Biosciences, Capital University of Science and Technology, Islamabad 44000, Pakistan; tahirmicrobiologist@gmail.com (M.T.K.); drshaukat@cust.edu.pk (S.I.M.)
[2] The State Key Laboratory of Microbial Metabolism, College of Life Sciences and Biotechnology, Shanghai Jiao Tong University, Shanghai 200240, China; amanbioinfo@gmail.com
[3] Department of Electrical Engineering, Capital University of Science and Technology, Islamabad 44000, Pakistan; aib@cust.edu.pk
[4] College of Life Sciences, Chongqing Normal University, Chongqing 401331, China; zhangyj@cqnu.edu.cn
[5] Department of Immunology and Microbiology, School of Medicine, Shanghai Jiao Tong University, Shanghai 200025, China; shulinzhang@sjtu.edu.cn (S.Z.); ajwei@sjtu.edu.cn (A.J.M.)
* Correspondence: dqwei@sjtu.edu.cn; Tel.: +86-21-3420-4573

Received: 16 August 2019; Accepted: 6 September 2019; Published: 26 September 2019

Abstract: Pyrazinamide (PZA) is the only drug for the elimination of latent *Mycobacterium tuberculosis* (MTB) isolates. However, due to the increased number of PZA-resistance, the chances of the success of global TB elimination seems to be more prolonged. Recently, marine natural products (MNPs) as an anti-TB agent have received much attention, where some compounds extracted from marine sponge, Haliclona sp. exhibited strong activity under aerobic and hypoxic conditions. In this study, we screened articles from 1994 to 2019 related to marine natural products (MNPs) active against latent MTB isolates. The literature was also mined for the major regulators to map them in the form of a pathway under the dormant stage. Five compounds were found to be more suitable that may be applied as an alternative to PZA for the better management of resistance under latent stage. However, the mechanism of actions behind these compounds is largely unknown. Here, we also applied synthetic biology to analyze the major regulatory pathway under latent TB that might be used for the screening of selective inhibitors among marine natural products (MNPs). We identified key regulators of MTB under latent TB through extensive literature mining and mapped them in the form of regulatory pathway, where SigH is negatively regulated by RshA. PknB, RshA, SigH, and RNA polymerase (RNA-pol) are the major regulators involved in MTB survival under latent stage. Further studies are needed to screen MNPs active against the main regulators of dormant MTB isolates. To reduce the PZA resistance burden, understanding the regulatory pathways may help in selective targets of MNPs from marine natural sources.

Keywords: marine anti-TB compounds; PZA; MTB; latent TB; sponges

1. Introduction

The latent state of tuberculosis (TB) is asymptomatic, but poses a risk in developing the active state of TB during the lifetime. According to the latest World Health Organization (WHO) report in 2018, TB is the leading public health problem among infectious diseases resulting from a single infectious agent, ahead of HIV/AIDS, and is the ninth leading cause of death worldwide. Approximately 1.3 million TB deaths occurred in 2017 excluding 374,000 deaths (10%) among HIV-positive individuals among 10.4 million total TB incidents (90% adults). About 1.7 billion people (23% of the world's population) are estimated to have a latent TB infection, indicating a risk of developing active TB during their lifetime. India, Indonesia, China, Philippines, and Pakistan are the top five countries comprising 56% of the world's estimated TB cases [1]. Among the infected individuals, 5–10% develop active TB. Such individuals suffer from latent TB, where the *Mycobacterium tuberculosis* (MTB) resides in alveolar macrophages in a non-replicative form (latent TB) [2–4]. The risk of developing active TB from non-replicative forms has been accounted in 10% of cases in latently infected populations [2,3,5], but may increase in cases of TB-HIV co-infections, immunosuppressive therapy, and old age [6–11]. Recently, a large number of studies reported drug resistances in TB [12–14] effecting the global TB control program.

1.1. PZA against Latent TB

Among the available anti-tuberculosis agents, pyrazinamide (PZA) is the only drug that is active against non-replicative MTB [15–18]. The host generates different types of stresses to eliminate the MTB isolates effectively. However, the organism switches a sensory system that generates a complex signaling network, assisting in entry into the latent state [19,19–22]. Before conversion into the latent stage, MTB faces a number of oxidoreductive stress in alveolar macrophages of the host including oxidative, acidic, and nitrative stress. These stresses are vital in the transition from active (replicative) TB into latent (non-replicative) state [23,24].

1.2. Signaling in Latent TB

The genome of MTB strains have diverse stress responders, switching on the genetic program for transition into latency [25,26]. Among these sensors under the latent stage are sigma (s) factors, which are the primary regulators of gene expression. MTB genomes encoded 13 factors of the sigma 70 family [27], which are categorized into four groups known as S1, 2, and 3 including SigA, SigB, and SigC, respectively, while the remaining one belongs to group 4, mainly involved in extra-cytoplasmic sensing and signaling [28–30]. These regulators have been called "S" factors due to their role in growth and stress conditions [28]. MTB senses redox through SigH, SigE, SigF, and SigL encoded regulators, playing a critical role in survival under extreme conditions [23,30,31]. Fernandes et al. first demonstrated that the role of SigH in oxidative stress [29] was also involved in the expression of thioredoxins (trxB1 and TrxC) and thioredoxin reductase, while the stress-responsive "S" factor and SigE helped mitigate oxidative stress. The "S" factor, along with SigB expression, is also regulated by SigE and SigH. [32,33]. Song et al. demonstrated that Rv3221a, an anti-sigma factor known as RshA in the same operon, [30] interacts with SigH at a 1:1 ratio [30], leading to SigH inhibition in vitro. Under oxidative stress, phosphorylation of RshA by PknB causes disruption of the RshA and SigH interactions, thereby regulating the induction of the oxidative stress response in mycobacteria [23].

1.3. Drugs Effective under Latent Stage

Pyrazinamide (PZA) is the only drug that kills MTB in a latent state, which has successfully reduced the time span of TB therapy from nine to six months [34–36]. PZA is a prodrug that depends on MTB encoded pyrazinamidase (PZase) (Figure 1A), whose activity is essential for the activation of PZA into the active form, pyrazinoic acid (POA). The POA targets ribosomal protein S1 (RpsA), aspartate decarboxylase (*panD*) (Figure 1D). The earlier protein helps in trans-translation while the latter is involved in ATP synthesis [37,38]. POA binds with RpsA, disrupting the complex of RpsA–tmRNA (Figure 1B). Recently, a large number of PZA-resistance cases have been reported, affecting the latent TB treatment. In our recent study, we evaluated the mechanism behind PZA-resistance in RpsA and PncA, showing a significant effect of mutation in PncA on protein activity [39–45]. Due to the large number of PZA-resistance cases, the latent stage of TB may function as a reservoir for transmission, affecting the global TB end control program.

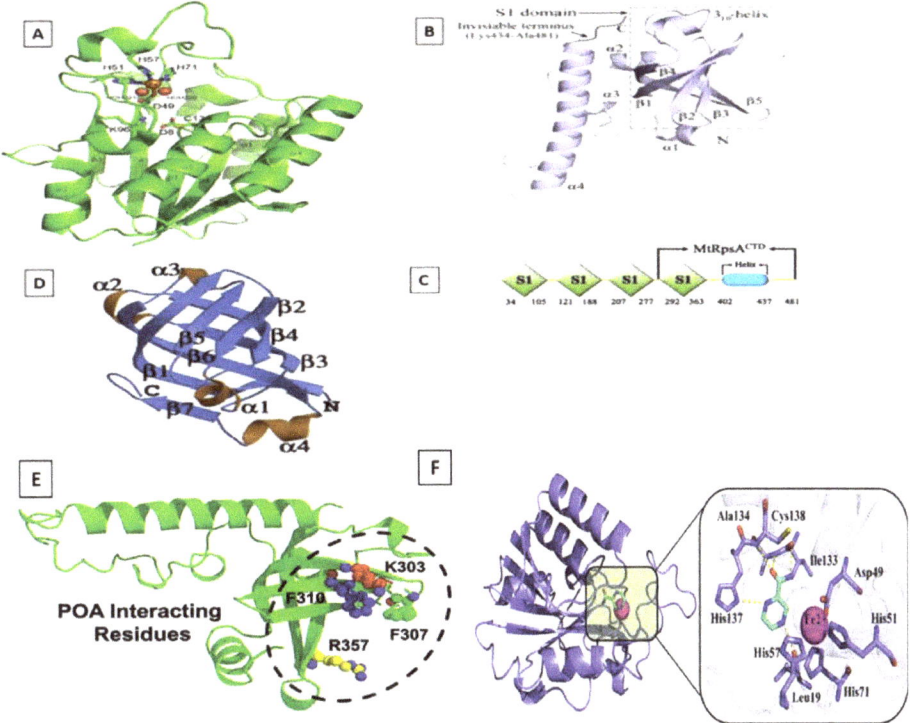

Figure 1. Crystal structures of PZA and POA targets. (**A**) PZase; (**B**) RpsA; (**C**) Domain organization of RpsA and its C-terminal domain (MtRpsACTD); (**D**) PanD. PZase converts PZA into POA inhibiting the activity of PanD and RpsA. POA interactions with RpsA (**E**) and PZA with PZase (**F**). The prodrug PZA is converted into active form, POA, inhibiting the trans-translational proteins (RpsA).

1.4. Marine Natural Products against Latent TB

With increased resistance to PZA, alternative novel bactericidal against non-replicating MTB will be important to reduce the transmission in the population and also for short period treatment. The screening for alternatives to PZA under latent TB from natural products is a validated approach. Here, nine out of 12 groups of available drugs are naturally derived [46]. Screening of more diverse natural product libraries has incentivized efforts in recent years [47]. The chemical diversity screening may be extended for marine natural products as more diverse and active products have been reported in marine environments [48]. Secondary metabolites that are produced by marine organisms have been found to be effective against many disease causing microorganisms [49]. Recently, some active compounds have been sourced from marine organisms against latent MTB isolates [47,50].

In a study by Felix et al. [51], a library of MNPs was screened where four among five compounds (Figure 2) were active against latent MTB isolates, containing 2 puupehenone group metabolites (Table 1). Propane,1,2-diol was not effective against dormant MTB isolates. These dormancy-active hits could reveal novel druggable targets under latent stage, and therefore may lead to an alternative of PZA.

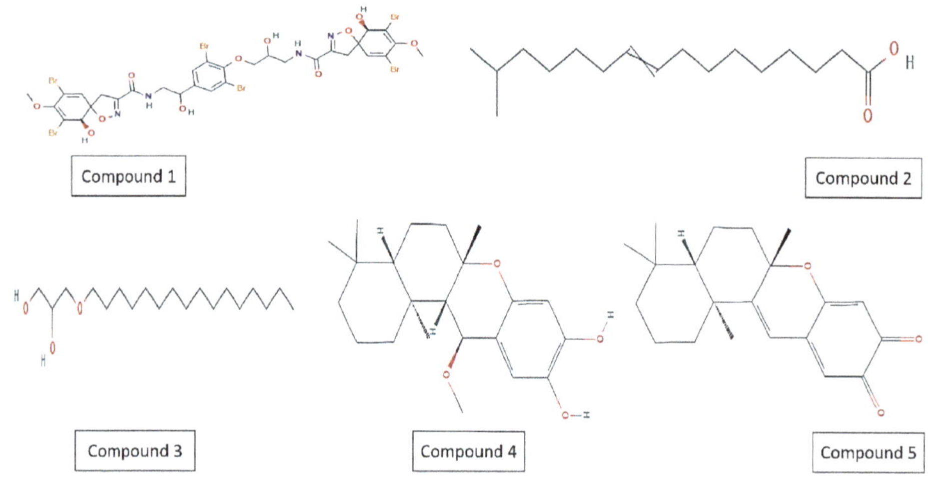

Figure 2. Compounds active against latent TB (dormant state). Compound 1, fistularin-3/11-epi-fistularin-3; compound 2, 15-methyl-9(Z)-hexadecenoic acid; compound 3, (hexadecyloxy) propane,1,2-diol; compound 4, 15- alpha methoxypuupehenol; and compound 5, puupehedione. Compound 3 exhibited mild activity against replicating MTB (active TB).

Table 1. Biological profile of marine pure compounds against dormant MTB isolates adopted from Felix et al; 2017 with permission from 2017 American Society for Microbiology [51].

Compound	Formula	Molecular Mass (kDa)	MIC_R (g/mL) [a]	MIC_D (g/mL) [b]	MIC_R/MIC_D	IC_{50} (g/mL)	SIR [c]	SID [d]	Source
1	C31H30Br6N4O11	1,114.02	8.5	Inactive	NA	200	23.5	NA	HBOI.047.F07
2	C19H40O3	316.53	60.8	22.5	2.7	200	3.3	8.5	HBOI.047.F07
3	C16H30O2	254.41	28.5	7.9	3.6	200	7.0	31.1	HBOI.031.C02
4	C22H32O4	360.49	11.3	0.5	21.8	8	0.7	15.5	HBOI.050.F04
5	C21H26O3	326.44	87.6	15.4	5.6	50.4	0.6	6.2	HBOI.050.F04

[a] MIC_R, MIC against replicating Mtb-Lux. [b] MIC_D, MIC against dormant Mtb-Lux. [c] SIR, SI for replicating Mtb-Lux. [d] SID, SI for dormant Mtb-Lux.

The core drug regimen has not been modified despite continuous efforts after a prolonged time [52]. Alternatively, research on MTB during in vivo has explored subpopulations of distinct metabolic states within a single host [53]. This knowledge may be useful to uncover the essential activities required for the survival of nonreplicating inhibition [54]. Whole cell screening under the dormancy–activating signaling pathway may provide a direct path to discovering novel bactericidals against latent MTB isolates. Here, the main goal of our study was to highlight the importance of marine drugs [55–57] that could effectively kill dormant bacteria as well as the analysis of some signaling pathways for more potent drug target identification.

2. Results

A total of 42 articles were retrieved from 1994 to 2018 containing data about the regulations and interactions of genes and proteins under latent MTB isolates where 14 manually searched papers also contained relevant information.

2.1. SigH Regulatory Network

We confirmed the interaction among the SigH regulons where a network file of "string" database in tsv format exposed different paths through Pathlinker of Cytoscape (Figures S2–S4). The stress responder, SigH, has a major role in controlling the response of pathogens to go into latent state and also in the survival of the pathogen. The regulatory pathway is shown in Figure 3A. The external stress signals are sensed by the membrane receptor protein PknB, initiating the signal transduction pathway by phosphorylating the SigH-RshA complex. This phosphorylation causes the disintegration of the SigH-RshA complex, allowing SigH to form a complex with RNA polymerase (RNA-pol), activating a series of stress responders. Upon activation, SigH and RshA are also synthesized, but RshA is continuously inactivated as long as the stress is sensed by PknB. The pathway is negatively regulated by RshA, while positively regulated by phosphorylated RshA (RshA-P), depending on the presence or absence of a stress signal (Figure 3A).

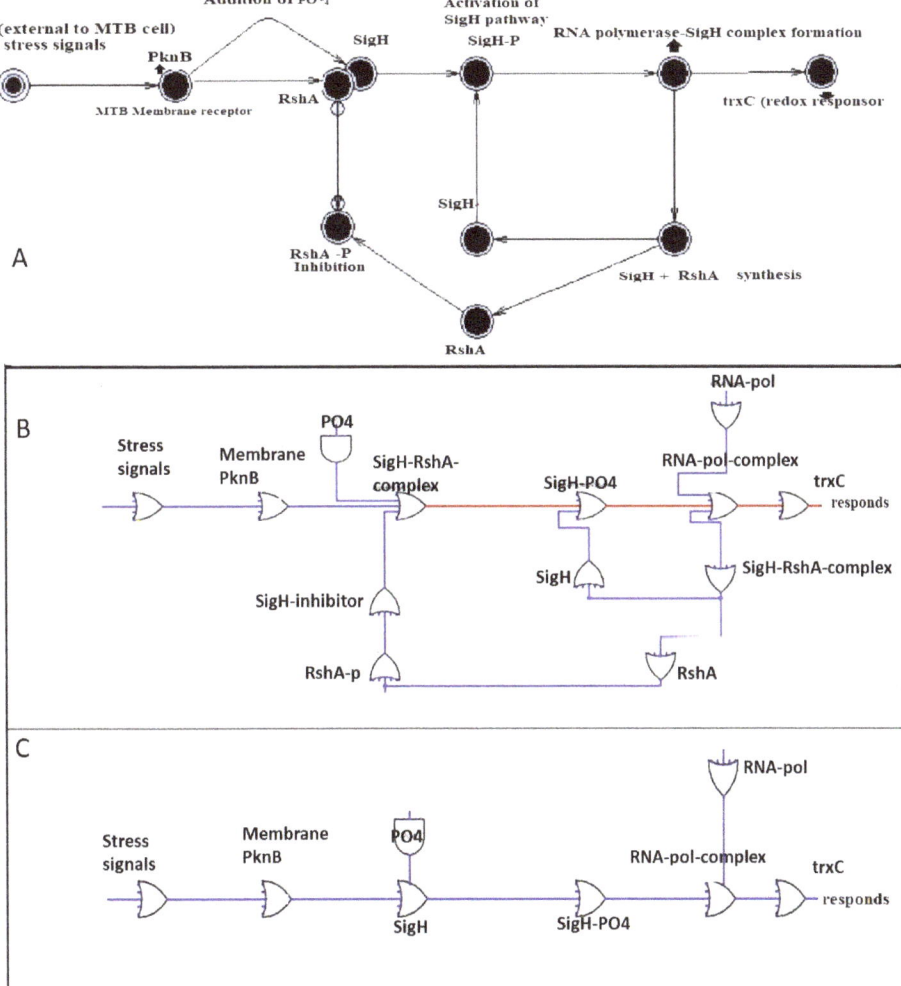

Figure 3. SigH signaling pathway under stress conditions. (**A**) The SigH signaling mechanism. (**B**) Boolean network simulation with the SigH-RshA complex negatively regulated the pathway, deactivating the regulatory pathway. (**C**) Boolean network simulation without the SigH-RshA complex, where the "SigH-PO$_4$" activates the mechanism. RshA-P: phosphorylated RshA; SigH-PO$_4$: phosphorylated SigH.

2.2. Paths Identification in the Network

All of the stress responders were used as input proteins and the interaction network was searched in a string database. The file (Figure S3) was imported into Cytoscape, where a total of 12 paths were identified using the Pathlinker plugin. The plugins computed multiple paths from the sources to targets where the longest path shown (Figure S1) was found to be most similar to the literature mapped SigH pathway (Figure 3A). The longest path linked all of the essential proteins regulated under the latent stage of MTB.

2.3. SigH Regulation and Marine Drugs

The interacting entities were subjected to six and nine different state stochastic simulations for 100 seconds in the active and inactive states to evaluate the dynamic behavior under latent state of MTB (Figure 3B,C). Stochastic simulations validate the desired functioning of the proposed biological regulatory systems (redox response) as shown in Figure 3. The SigH regulatory pathway may play a crucial role in the survival of the pathogen under extreme stress environment.

3. Discussion

Currently, PZA is the only drug regularly prescribed along with other first-line drugs for the effective control of dormant MTB and is recommended in sensitive as well as multi and extensive drug resistance. However, due to an increased number of PZA-resistance, alternative sources of natural products that are active against the dormant isolate in acidic pH are continuously being sought. Sponges in the marine environment are rich sources of such compounds. Quinones with high selectivity against dormant MTB are from a sponge from the Petrosia (Strongylophora) genus. Terpene quinones including puupehenone metabolites have been extensively studied for their antimicrobial and cytotoxic properties [58–60]. The puupehenone derivatives showed anti-TB activity as reported earlier [50]. The MIC of 15-methoxypuupehenol was 20-fold lower and effective against dormant, but not replicating. Puupehedione and Puupehenone had been previously extracted from the sponge Hyrtios sp. [58]. Puupehedione had minor activity against replicating MTB [50], however, a 6-fold selectivity of puupehedione against dormant MTB was still observed.

Puupehenone metabolites inhibit NADH oxidase activity in submitochondrial particles [61,62]. Weinstein et al. observed a bactericidal effect for M. tuberculosis's type II NADH oxidase (NDH-2) inhibitors in a murine model [63,64]. Inhibitors of NDH-2 proteins such as thioridazine, exhibited bactericidal activity against dormant MTB when compared to replicating isolates [65]. The synthesis of puupehenone enables a path for these molecules [66]. Characterization of the molecular targets for these antimycobacterial marine natural products with selective activity against dormant MTB will be helpful for exploring the insight mechanisms of the survival of dormant MTB under the latent stage of infections.

The halicyclamine alkaloids (HA) with piperidine rings, haliclonacyclamines A and B (Figure 2) C-1 and C-2 [67], 22-hydroxyhaliclonacyclamine B (C-3) [68], and halicyclamine A (C-4) (Figure 4) [69] have been discovered from the marine sponge Haliclona sp. [70]. Haliclona sp. is one among the dominant sponges at Heron Island, occurring at depths of about 15 m in reef slope [71]. The anti-TB bactericidal and bacteriostatic activity of C-3 and C-4 were evaluated under aerobic and hypoxic conditions. The colony forming unit (CFUs) of M. bovis BCG was not detected after eight days and 10 days of incubation under aerobic and hypoxic environment, respectively, indicating bactericidal activity of C-2. Compound C-4 exhibited a strong cidal effect against mycobacterium sp. including M. tuberculosis H37Ra (MICs of 2.16–10.82 µM) under dormant state. Compounds C-1 and C-2 also exhibited cidal activities against replicating and non-replicating (latent state) of MTB. C-3 exhibited weak activity that might be due to the 22-hydroxy group. Compound C-4, which is involved in catalytic conversion of inosine monophosphate to xanthosine monophosphate in the de novo synthesis of guanine nucleotides, was isolated as an inhibitor of inosine 5′-monophosphate dehydrogenase

(IMPDH) [69]. IMPDH was cloned into M. smegmatis to study the anti-TB mechanism. However, both the wild-type M. smegmatis and IMPDH over-expressing strains exhibited similar MIC values, indicating that IMPDH was not the target of compound C-4 [70]. Another HA, neopetrosiamine A (C-5) (Figure 2), isolated from sponge Neopetrosia proxima growing near Puerto Rico in a marine environment [72], showed good cidal activity against MTB H37Rv (MIC:17.05 μM).

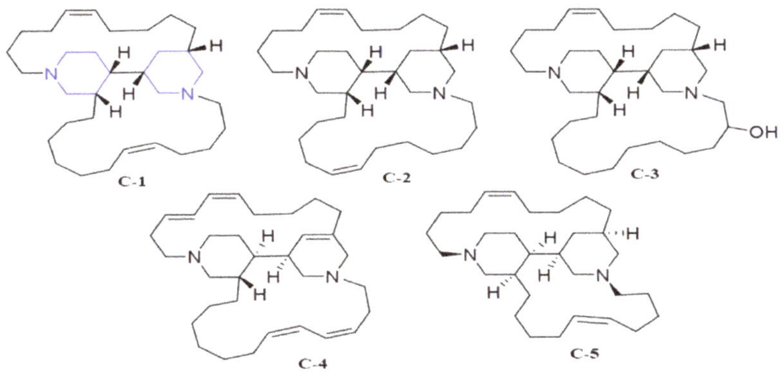

Figure 4. Anti-TB compounds, C-1 to C-5 active against latent TB. The blue colored lines were the same in all compounds. Haliclonacyclamines A and B (C-1 and C-2). 22-hydroxyhaliclonacyclamine B (C-3), Halicyclamine A (C-4), and neopetrosiamine A (C-5).

The stress response under the latent state of MTB is mediated by many regulatory genes and the role of SigH in the oxidative stress was first established by Fernandes et al. [29] through experiments using *M. smegmatis* SigH mutants. SigH is a major MTB regulator that provides protection from reactive oxygen species generated by the human host [31,73]. The SigH-encoded protein protects MTB against oxidative stress by regulating the expression of the stress-responsive factors SigE and thioredoxins trxB1 and trxC. The stress-responsive "S" factor and SigB were also regulated by the SigE and SigH regulators. However, the mechanism of SigH regulation was not clearly explored, and neither were there any synthetic biology approaches applied for better understanding. Marine compounds shown in Figure 2 may be applied against dormant isolates to find their effect. Furthermore, the mechanism may also be through a knockout system.

Prokaryotic RNA-pol may be a potent target as it plays a role in the initiation of the complex network. RNA-pol is directed by sigma factors toward specific promotors through the formation of a sigma/RNA-pol holoenzyme, which may be a closed stable complex that is ineffectual for transcription initiation (sigma 54), or may proceed directly to an open complex that is capable of transcription (sigma 70). RNA-pol is an ideal drug target for a number of antibiotics because it is an integral part of a crucial cellular process [74,75].

4. Methods

4.1. Literature Search

To map a signaling pathway under the latent stage of MTB, the RISmed package of R was used to retrieve relevant literature from the Entrez Utilities to the PubMed database at National Center For Biotechnology Information (NCBI) [76–78]. The RISmed package is fast and time efficient, extracting the exact information. The key words, latent stage TB, dormant state MTB, MTB survival under stress, role of sigma factors, SigH of MTB, regulation of MTB pathway under stress condition, RshA role, role of TrxC, PknB, and stress regulation were used to mine the relevant information from the literature databases. Subsequently, all the relevant papers were manually searched for the genes and proteins expressed under the latent stage.

4.2. Pathway Construction Using Systems Biology Approach

All the major regulators involved in signaling and interactions were extracted from the literature and mapped in the form of a regulatory network in UPPAAL, an integrated tool for modeling [79], in the form of a pathway.

4.3. Validation of SigH Regulatory Pathway

The SigH regulatory pathway mapped from the literature was further confirmed for their interactions in a "STRING" database [80]. All the SigH regulons were entered as input in the string database to observe the interacting network. The protein network was further increased by the addition of more nodes (proteins) until all of the extracted entities were found to be interconnected in a single network. The network file was downloaded in the Tab Separated Values (TSV) format (Table S1) and imported into Cytoscape v 3.5.1 [81] where different paths were generated inside the network using the Pathlinker [82] plugin in Cytoscape. The sources and targets were selected based on the mined literature data, and the longest path was searched using a background protein interaction network. Pathlinker requires three inputs: a (directed) network G, a set S of "sources", and a set T of "targets". Each element of S and T must be a node in G. Pathlinker efficiently computes several short paths from the receptors to transcriptional regulators (TRs) in a network and can accurately rebuild an inclusive set of signaling pathways from the NetPath and KEGG databases. Pathlinker has a higher precision and recall when compared to several state-of-the-art algorithms. The longest path was analyzed based on the score of Pathlinker using the ANIMO plugin [83] for visualization purposes.

4.4. Synthetic Biology and SigH Activation

The pathway was simulated for 100 s using the Java Script [84] to analyze the effect on the active and inactive state of SigH regulation.

5. Conclusions

The marine environment, a highly valuable source for new lead structures, is a rich source of anti-TB bioactive compounds that have the potential to be used as an alternative to PZA. The biological activity of these leads gives hope for effective anti-TB agents that will show low-toxicity under the latent stage. Here in this review, we highlighted some marine natural products that are effective against latent TB. Furthermore, we mapped a novel SigH regulatory pathway whose regulons may be patent targets to verify the mechanism of action. Although studies have been carried out to discover these agents, the mechanism of action is still uncertain and will require future research. These compounds may be tested against the potent targets of the SigH signaling pathway, which is required for the survival of MTB under different kinds of stress including oxidative and acidic stress. This study provides useful information about the screening of marine natural products active against latent TB that may be tested against the signaling pathway under the latent stage of MTB.

Supplementary Materials: The following are available online at http://www.mdpi.com/1660-3397/17/10/549/s1, Figure S1: Longest path generated through the Cytoscape plugin, Pathlinker; Figure S2: Pathlinker identified paths in a string network file; Figure S3: PknB and SigH network generated in string; Figure S4: PknB, SigH, and RshA containing network in the string database. Table S1: PknB and SigH network.

Author Contributions: D.Q.W., A.I.B., and S.I.M. designed and analyzed the project. A.I.B., M.T.K., A.J.W., and A.C.K. performed the experiment and wrote manuscript. S.Z. and Y.-J.Z. analyzed the data and revised the manuscript.

Funding: This work was supported by grants from the Key Research Area Grant 2016YFA0501703 of the Ministry of Science and Technology of China, the National Natural Science Foundation of China (Contract no. 61832019, 61503244), and the State Key Lab of Microbial Metabolism and Joint Research Funds for Medical and Engineering and Scientific Research at Shanghai Jiao Tong University (YG2017ZD14).

Acknowledgments: We would like to thank Sahar Fazal, Head of Bioinformatics and Biosciences department for their technical support.

Conflicts of Interest: The authors declare no conflict of interest.

References

1. WHO. Global Tuberculosis Report 2017. Available online: http://apps.who.int/medicinedocs/en/m/abstract/Js23360en/ (accessed on 6 September 2019).
2. Ai, J.W.; Ruan, Q.L.; Liu, Q.H.; Zhang, W.H. Updates on the risk factors for latent tuberculosis reactivation and their managements. *Emerg. Microbes Infect.* **2016**, *5*, e10. [CrossRef] [PubMed]
3. Esmail, H.; Barry, C.E.; Wilkinson, R.J. Understanding latent tuberculosis: The key to improved diagnostic and novel treatment strategies. *Drug Discov. Today* **2012**, *17*, 514–521. [CrossRef] [PubMed]
4. Houben, R.M.G.J.; Dodd, P.J. The Global Burden of Latent Tuberculosis Infection: A Re-estimation Using Mathematical Modelling. *PLoS Med.* **2016**, *13*, e1002152. [CrossRef] [PubMed]
5. Fogel, N. Tuberculosis: A disease without boundaries. *Tuberculosis* **2015**, *95*, 527–531. [CrossRef] [PubMed]
6. Bruchfeld, J.; Correia-Neves, M.; Källenius, G. Tuberculosis and HIV Coinfection. *Cold Spring Harb. Perspect. Med.* **2015**, *5*. [CrossRef] [PubMed]
7. Fujita, A. Tuberculosis in HIV/AIDS Patients. *Nihon Rinsho* **2017**, *69*, 1433–1437.
8. Mekonnen, D.; Derbie, A.; Desalegn, E. TB/HIV co-infections and associated factors among patients on directly observed treatment short course in Northeastern Ethiopia: A 4 years retrospective study. *BMC Res. Notes* **2015**, *8*. [CrossRef] [PubMed]
9. Pawlowski, A.; Jansson, M.; Sköld, M.; Rottenberg, M.E.; Källenius, G. Tuberculosis and HIV Co-Infection. *PLoS Pathog.* **2012**, *8*. [CrossRef]
10. Schutz, C.; Meintjes, G.; Almajid, F.; Wilkinson, R.J.; Pozniak, A. Clinical management of tuberculosis and HIV-1 co-infection. *Eur. Respir. J.* **2010**, *36*, 1460–1481. [CrossRef]
11. Tesfaye, B.; Alebel, A.; Gebrie, A.; Zegeye, A.; Tesema, C.; Kassie, B. The twin epidemics: Prevalence of TB/HIV co-infection and its associated factors in Ethiopia; A systematic review and meta-analysis. *PLoS ONE* **2018**, *13*, e0203986. [CrossRef]
12. Anand, R. Identification of Potential Antituberculosis Drugs Through Docking and Virtual Screening. *Interdiscip. Sci. Comput. Life Sci.* **2018**, *10*, 419–429. [CrossRef] [PubMed]
13. Hosen, M.I.; Tanmoy, A.M.; Mahbuba, D.A.; Salma, U.; Nazim, M.; Islam, M.T.; Akhteruzzaman, S. Application of a subtractive genomics approach for in silico identification and characterization of novel drug targets in Mycobacterium tuberculosis F11. *Interdiscip. Sci. Comput. Life Sci.* **2014**, *6*, 48–56. [CrossRef] [PubMed]
14. Durairaj, D.R.; Shanmughavel, P. In Silico Drug Design of Thiolactomycin Derivatives Against Mtb-KasA Enzyme to Inhibit Multidrug Resistance of Mycobacterium tuberculosis. *Interdiscip. Sci. Comput. Life Sci.* **2019**, *11*, 215–225. [CrossRef] [PubMed]
15. Alexander, D.C.; Ma, J.H.; Guthrie, J.L.; Blair, J.; Chedore, P.; Jamieson, F.B. Gene sequencing for routine verification of pyrazinamide resistance in Mycobacterium tuberculosis: A role for pncA but not rpsA. *J. Clin. Microbiol.* **2012**, *50*, 3726–3728. [CrossRef] [PubMed]
16. Allana, S.; Shashkina, E.; Mathema, B.; Bablishvili, N.; Tukvadze, N.; Shah, N.S.; Kempker, R.R.; Blumberg, H.M.; Moodley, P.; Mlisana, K.; et al. pncA Gene Mutations Associated with Pyrazinamide Resistance in Drug-Resistant Tuberculosis, South Africa and Georgia. *Emerg. Infect. Dis.* **2017**, *23*, 491–495. [CrossRef] [PubMed]
17. Aono, A.; Chikamatsu, K.; Yamada, H.; Kato, T.; Mitarai, S. Association between pncA gene mutations, pyrazinamidase activity, and pyrazinamide susceptibility testing in Mycobacterium tuberculosis. *Antimicrob. Agents Chemother.* **2014**, *58*, 4928–4930. [CrossRef] [PubMed]
18. Khan, M.T.; Malik, S.I.; Ali, S.; Sheed Khan, A.; Nadeem, T.; Zeb, M.T.; Masood, N.; Afzal, M.T. Prevalence of Pyrazinamide Resistance in Khyber Pakhtunkhwa, Pakistan. *Microb. Drug Resist.* **2018**. [CrossRef] [PubMed]
19. Black, G.F.; Thiel, B.A.; Ota, M.O.; Parida, S.K.; Adegbola, R.; Boom, W.H.; Dockrell, H.M.; Franken, K.L.M.C.; Friggen, A.H.; Hill, P.C.; et al. Immunogenicity of novel DosR regulon-encoded candidate antigens of Mycobacterium tuberculosis in three high-burden populations in Africa. *Clin. Vaccine Immunol. CVI* **2009**, *16*, 1203–1212. [CrossRef]

20. Hatzios, S.K.; Baer, C.E.; Rustad, T.R.; Siegrist, M.S.; Pang, J.M.; Ortega, C.; Alber, T.; Grundner, C.; Sherman, D.R.; Bertozzi, C.R. Osmosensory signaling in Mycobacterium tuberculosis mediated by a eukaryotic-like Ser/Thr protein kinase. *Proc. Natl. Acad. Sci. USA* **2013**, *110*, E5069–E5077. [CrossRef]

21. Honaker, R.; Dhiman, R.; Narayanasamy, P.; Crick, D.; Voskuil, M. DosS responds to a reduced electron transport system to induce the Mycobacterium tuberculosis DosR regulon. *J. Bacteriol.* **2010**, *192*, 6447–6455. [CrossRef]

22. Sherman, D.; Voskuil, M.; Schnappinger, D.; Liao, R.; Harrell, M.; Schoolnik, G.; Park, H.; Guinn, K.; Voskuil, M.; Tompa, M.; et al. Regulation of the Mycobacterium tuberculosis hypoxic response gene encoding alpha-crystallin. *Proc. Natl. Acad. Sci. USA* **2001**, *98*, 7534–7539. [CrossRef] [PubMed]

23. Park, S.T.; Kang, C.M.; Husson, R.N. Regulation of the SigH stress response regulon by an essential protein kinase in Mycobacterium tuberculosis. *Proc. Natl. Acad. Sci. USA* **2008**, *105*, 13105–13110. [CrossRef] [PubMed]

24. Busche, T.; Šilar, R.; Pičmanová, M.; Pátek, M.; Kalinowski, J. Transcriptional regulation of the operon encoding stress-responsive ECF sigma factor SigH and its anti-sigma factor RshA, and control of its regulatory network in Corynebacterium glutamicum. *BMC Genom.* **2012**, *13*, 445. [CrossRef] [PubMed]

25. Kumar, A.; Farhana, A.; Guidry, L.; Saini, V.; Hondalus, M.; Steyn, A.J. Redox homeostasis in mycobacteria: The key to tuberculosis control? *Expert Rev. Mol. Med.* **2011**, *13*, e39. [CrossRef] [PubMed]

26. Trivedi, A.; Singh, N.; Bhat, S.A.; Gupta, P.; Kumar, A. Redox biology of tuberculosis pathogenesis. *Adv. Microb. Physiol.* **2012**, *60*, 263–324. [PubMed]

27. Cole, S.T.; Brosch, R.; Parkhill, J.; Garnier, T.; Churcher, C.; Harris, D.; Gordon, S.V.; Eiglmeier, K.; Gas, S.; Barry, C.E., 3rd. Deciphering the biology of Mycobacterium tuberculosis from the complete genome sequence. *Nature* **1998**, *393*, 537–544. [CrossRef] [PubMed]

28. Bashyam, M.; Hasnain, S. The extracytoplasmic function sigma factors: Role in bacterial pathogenesis. *Infect. Genet. Evol.* **2004**, *4*, 301–308. [CrossRef] [PubMed]

29. Fernandes, N.D.; Wu, Q.L.; Kong, D.; Puyang, X.; Garg, S.; Husson, R.N. A mycobacterial extracytoplasmic sigma factor involved in survival following heat shock and oxidative stress. *J. Bacteriol.* **1999**, *181*, 4266–4274.

30. Song, T.; Dove, S.L.; Lee, K.H.; Husson, R.N. RshA, an anti-sigma factor that regulates the activity of the mycobacterial stress response sigma factor SigH. *Mol. Microbiol.* **2003**, *50*, 949–959. [CrossRef]

31. Raman, S.; Song, T.; Puyang, X.; Bardarov, S.; Jacobs, J.; Husson, R.N. The alternative sigma factor sigh regulates major components of oxidative and heat stress responses in Mycobacterium tuberculosis. *J. Bacteriol.* **2001**, *183*, 6119–6125. [CrossRef]

32. Graham, J.E.; Clark-Curtiss, J.E. Identification of Mycobacterium tuberculosis RNAs synthesized in response to phagocytosis by human macrophages by selective capture of transcribed sequences (SCOTS). *Proc. Natl. Acad. Sci. USA* **1999**, *96*, 11554–11559. [CrossRef] [PubMed]

33. Kaushal, D.; Schroeder, B.G.; Tyagi, S.; Yoshimatsu, T.; Scott, C.; Ko, C.; Carpenter, L.; Mehrotra, J.; Manabe, Y.C.; Fleischmann, R.D.; et al. Reduced immunopathology and mortality despite tissue persistence in a Mycobacterium tuberculosis mutant lacking alternative sigma factor, SigH. *Proc. Natl. Acad. Sci. USA* **2002**, *99*, 8330–8335. [CrossRef] [PubMed]

34. Mitchison, D.A. The action of antituberculosis drugs in short-course chemotherapy. *Tubercle* **1985**, *66*, 219–225. [CrossRef]

35. Yang, J.; Liu, Y.; Bi, J.; Cai, Q.; Liao, X.; Li, W.; Guo, C.; Zhang, Q.; Lin, T.; Zhao, Y.; et al. Structural basis for targeting the ribosomal protein S1 of Mycobacterium tuberculosis by pyrazinamide. *Mol. Microbiol.* **2015**, *95*, 791–803. [CrossRef] [PubMed]

36. Yadon, A.N.; Maharaj, K.; Adamson, J.H.; Lai, Y.-P.; Sacchettini, J.C.; Ioerger, T.R.; Rubin, E.J.; Pym, A.S. A comprehensive characterization of PncA polymorphisms that confer resistance to pyrazinamide. *Nat. Commun.* **2017**, *8*. [CrossRef] [PubMed]

37. Lu, P.; Haagsma, A.C.; Pham, H.; Maaskant, J.J.; Mol, S.; Lill, H.; Bald, D. Pyrazinoic Acid Decreases the Proton Motive Force, Respiratory ATP Synthesis Activity, and Cellular ATP Levels. *Antimicrob. Agents Chemother.* **2011**, *55*, 5354–5357. [CrossRef]

38. Ying, Z.; Wade, M.M.; Scorpio, A.; Zhang, H.; Sun, Z. Mode of action of pyrazinamide: Disruption of Mycobacterium tuberculosis membrane transport and energetics by pyrazinoic acid. *J. Antimicrob. Chemother.* **2003**, *52*, 790–795.

39. Khan, M.T.; Malik, S.I. Structural dynamics behind variants in pyrazinamidase and pyrazinamide resistance. *J. Biomol. Struct. Dyn.* **2019**, 1–15. [CrossRef]

40. Khan, M. Pyrazinamide resistance and mutations L19R, R140H, and E144K in Pyrazinamidase of Mycobacterium tuberculosis. *J. Cell. Biochem.* **2019**, *120*, 7154–7166. [CrossRef]

41. Khan, M.T.; Khan, A.; Rehman, A.U.; Wang, Y.; Akhtar, K.; Malik, S.I.; Wei, D.Q. Structural and free energy landscape of novel mutations in ribosomal protein S1 (rpsA) associated with pyrazinamide resistance. *Sci. Rep.* **2019**, *9*, 7482. [CrossRef]

42. Khan, M.T.; Rehaman, A.U.; Junaid, M.; Malik, S.I.; Wei, D.Q. Insight into novel clinical mutants of RpsA-S324F, E325K, and G341R of Mycobacterium tuberculosis associated with pyrazinamide resistance. *Comput. Struct. Biotechnol. J.* **2018**, *16*, 379–387. [CrossRef] [PubMed]

43. Junaid, M.; Khan, M.T.; Malik, S.I.; Wei, D.Q. Insights into the mechanisms of pyrazinamide resistance of three pyrazinamidase mutants N11K, P69T and D126N. *J. Chem. Inf. Model.* **2018**. [CrossRef] [PubMed]

44. Rehman, A.U.; Khan, M.T.; Liu, H.; Wadood, A.; Malik, S.I.; Chen, H.-F. Exploring the Pyrazinamide Drug Resistance Mechanism of Clinical Mutants T370P and W403G in Ribosomal Protein S1 of Mycobacterium tuberculosis. *J. Chem. Inf. Model.* **2019**, *59*, 1584–1597. [CrossRef] [PubMed]

45. Khan, M.T.; Malik, S.I.; Bhatti, A.I.; Ali, S.; Khan, A.S.; Zeb, M.T.; Nadeem, T.; Fazal, S. Pyrazinamide-resistant mycobacterium tuberculosis isolates from Khyber Pakhtunkhwa and rpsA mutations. *J. Biol. Regul. Homeost. Agents* **2018**, *32*, 705–709. [PubMed]

46. Newman, D.J.; Cragg, G.M. Natural Products as Sources of New Drugs from 1981 to 2014. *J. Nat. Prod.* **2016**, *79*, 629–661. [CrossRef] [PubMed]

47. Farah, S.I.; Abdelrahman, A.A.; North, E.J.; Chauhan, H. Opportunities and Challenges for Natural Products as Novel Antituberculosis Agents. *Assay Drug Dev. Technol.* **2016**, *14*, 29–38. [CrossRef] [PubMed]

48. Montaser, R.; Luesch, H. Marine natural products: A new wave of drugs? *Future Med. Chem.* **2011**, *3*, 1475–1489. [CrossRef]

49. Hughes, C.C.; Fenical, W. Antibacterials from the Sea. *Chemistry* **2010**, *16*, 12512–12525. [CrossRef]

50. Hou, X.-M.; Wang, C.-Y.; Gerwick, W.H.; Shao, C.-L. Marine natural products as potential anti-tubercular agents. *Eur. J. Med. Chem.* **2019**, *165*, 273–292. [CrossRef]

51. Felix, C.R.; Gupta, R.; Geden, S.; Roberts, J.; Winder, P.; Pomponi, S.A.; Diaz, M.C.; Reed, J.K.; Wright, A.E.; Rohde, K.H. Selective Killing of Dormant Mycobacterium tuberculosis by Marine Natural Products. *Antimicrob. Agents Chemother.* **2017**, *61*, e00743-17. [CrossRef]

52. Zumla, A.; Nahid, P.; Cole, S.T. Advances in the development of new tuberculosis drugs and treatment regimens. *Nat. Rev. Drug Discov.* **2013**, *12*, 388–404. [CrossRef] [PubMed]

53. Dhar, N.; McKinney, J.; Manina, G. Phenotypic Heterogeneity in Mycobacterium tuberculosis. *Microbiol. Spectr.* **2016**, *4* [CrossRef]

54. Koul, A.; Arnoult, E.; Lounis, N.; Guillemont, J.; Andries, K. The challenge of new drug discovery for tuberculosis. *Nature* **2011**, *469*, 483–490. [CrossRef] [PubMed]

55. McCulloch, M.W.B.; Haltli, B.; Marchbank, D.H.; Kerr, R.G. Evaluation of pseudopteroxazole and pseudopterosin derivatives against Mycobacterium tuberculosis and other pathogens. *Mar. Drugs* **2012**, *10*, 1711–1728. [CrossRef] [PubMed]

56. Canché Chay, C.I.; Gómez Cansino, R.; Espitia Pinzón, C.I.; Torres-Ochoa, R.O.; Martínez, R. Synthesis and anti-tuberculosis activity of the marine natural product caulerpin and its analogues. *Mar. Drugs* **2014**, *12*, 1757–1772. [CrossRef] [PubMed]

57. Braña, A.F.; Sarmiento-Vizcaíno, A.; Pérez-Victoria, I.; Martín, J.; Otero, L.; Palacios-Gutiérrez, J.J.; Fernández, J.; Mohamedi, Y.; Fontanil, T.; Salmón, M.; et al. Desertomycin G, a New Antibiotic with Activity against Mycobacterium tuberculosis and Human Breast Tumor Cell Lines Produced by Streptomyces althioticus MSM3, Isolated from the Cantabrian Sea Intertidal Macroalgae Ulva sp. *Mar. Drugs* **2019**, *17*, 114. [CrossRef] [PubMed]

58. Bourguet-Kondracki, M.L.; Lacombe, F.; Guyot, M. Methanol adduct of puupehenone, a biologically active derivative from the marine sponge Hyrtios species. *J. Nat. Prod.* **1999**, *62*, 1304–1305. [CrossRef]

59. Hagiwara, K.; Garcia Hernandez, J.E.; Harper, M.K.; Carroll, A.; Motti, C.A.; Awaya, J.; Nguyen, H.-Y.; Wright, A.D. Puupehenol, a potent antioxidant antimicrobial meroterpenoid from a Hawaiian deep-water Dactylospongia sp. sponge. *J. Nat. Prod.* **2015**, *78*, 325–329. [CrossRef]

60. Gordaliza, M. Cytotoxic terpene quinones from marine sponges. *Mar. Drugs* **2010**, *8*, 2849–2870. [CrossRef]

61. Ciavatta, M.L.; Lopez Gresa, M.P.; Gavagnin, M.; Romero, V.; Melck, D.; Manzo, E.; Guo, Y.-W.; van Soest, R.; Cimino, G. Studies on puupehenone-metabolites of a Dysidea sp.: Structure and biological activity. *Tetrahedron* **2007**, *63*, 1380–1384. [CrossRef]

62. Robinson, S.J.; Hoobler, E.K.; Riener, M.; Loveridge, S.T.; Tenney, K.; Valeriote, F.A.; Holman, T.R.; Crews, P. Using enzyme assays to evaluate the structure and bioactivity of sponge-derived meroterpenes. *J. Nat. Prod.* **2009**, *72*, 1857–1863. [CrossRef] [PubMed]

63. Weinstein, E.A.; Yano, T.; Li, L.-S.; Avarbock, D.; Avarbock, A.; Helm, D.; McColm, A.A.; Duncan, K.; Lonsdale, J.T.; Rubin, H. Inhibitors of type II NADH: Menaquinone oxidoreductase represent a class of antitubercular drugs. *Proc. Natl. Acad. Sci. USA* **2005**, *102*, 4548–4553. [CrossRef] [PubMed]

64. Awasthy, D.; Ambady, A.; Narayana, A.; Morayya, S.; Sharma, U. Roles of the two type II NADH dehydrogenases in the survival of Mycobacterium tuberculosis in vitro. *Gene* **2014**, *550*, 110–116. [CrossRef] [PubMed]

65. Rao, S.P.S.; Alonso, S.; Rand, L.; Dick, T.; Pethe, K. The protonmotive force is required for maintaining ATP homeostasis and viability of hypoxic, nonreplicating Mycobacterium tuberculosis. *Proc. Natl. Acad. Sci. USA* **2008**, *105*, 11945–11950. [CrossRef] [PubMed]

66. Kraus, G.A.; Nguyen, T.; Bae, J.; Hostetter, J.; Steadham, E. Synthesis and antitubercular activity of tricyclic analogs of puupehenone. *Tetrahedron* **2004**, *60*, 4223–4225. [CrossRef]

67. Clark, R.J.; Field, K.L.; Charan, R.D.; Garson, M.J.; Brereton, M.; Willis, A.C. The haliclonacyclamines, cytotoxic tertiary alkaloids from the tropical marine sponge Haliclona sp. *Tetrahedron* **1998**, *54*, 8811–8826. [CrossRef]

68. Arai, M.; Ishida, S.; Setiawan, A.; Kobayashi, M. Haliclonacyclamines, tetracyclic alkylpiperidine alkaloids, as anti-dormant mycobacterial substances from a marine sponge of Haliclona sp. *Chem. Pharm. Bull. (Tokyo)* **2009**, *57*, 1136–1138. [CrossRef]

69. Jaspars, M.; Pasupathy, V.; Crews, P. A tetracyclic diamine alkaloid, halicyclamine A, from the marine sponge Haliclona sp. *J. Org. Chem.* **1994**, *59*, 3253–3255. [CrossRef]

70. Arai, M.; Sobou, M.; Vilchéze, C.; Baughn, A.; Hashizume, H.; Pruksakorn, P.; Ishida, S.; Matsumoto, M.; Jacobs, W.R.; Kobayashi, M. Halicyclamine A, a marine spongean alkaloid as a lead for anti-tuberculosis agent. *Bioorg. Med. Chem.* **2008**, *16*, 6732–6736. [CrossRef]

71. Garson, M.J.; Flowers, A.E.; Webb, R.I.; Charan, R.D.; McCaffrey, E.J. A sponge/dinoflagellate association in the haplosclerid sponge Haliclona sp.: Cellular origin of cytotoxic alkaloids by percoll density gradient fractionation. *Cell Tissue Res.* **1998**, *293*, 365–373. [CrossRef]

72. Wei, X.; Nieves, K.; Rodríguez, A.D. Neopetrosiamine A, biologically active bis-piperidine alkaloid from the Caribbean sea sponge Neopetrosia proxima. *Bioorg. Med. Chem. Lett.* **2010**, *20*, 5905–5908. [CrossRef] [PubMed]

73. Manganelli, R.; Voskuil, M.I.; Schoolnik, G.K.; Dubnau, E.; Gomez, M.; Smith, I. Role of the extracytoplasmic-function sigma factor sigma(H) in Mycobacterium tuberculosis global gene expression. *Mol. Microbiol.* **2002**, *45*, 365–374. [CrossRef] [PubMed]

74. Campbell, E.A.; Korzheva, N.; Mustaev, A.; Murakami, K.; Nair, S.; Goldfarb, A.; Darst, S.A. Structural mechanism for rifampicin inhibition of bacterial rna polymerase. *Cell* **2001**, *104*, 901–912. [CrossRef]

75. Ghosh, T.; Bose, D.; Zhang, X. Mechanisms for activating bacterial RNA polymerase. *FEMS Microbiol. Rev.* **2010**, *34*, 611–627. [CrossRef] [PubMed]

76. Vuorre, M. Quantitative Literature Review with R: Exploring Psychonomic Society Journals, Part I. Available online: https://vuorre.netlify.com/post/2017/quantitative-literature-review-with-r-part-i/ (accessed on 9 October 2018).

77. Rani, J.; Shah, A.B.R.; Ramachandran, S. pubmed.mineR: An R package with text-mining algorithms to analyse PubMed abstracts. *J. Biosci.* **2015**, *40*, 671–682. [CrossRef]

78. RISmed: Download Content from NCBI Databases Version 2.1.7 from CRAN. Available online: https://rdrr.io/cran/RISmed/ (accessed on 9 October 2018).

79. Larsen, K.G.; Mikucionis, M.; Nielsen, B.; Skou, A. Testing Real-time Embedded Software Using UPPAAL-TRON: An Industrial Case Study. In Proceedings of the 5th ACM International Conference on Embedded Software 2005, Jersey City, NJ, USA, 18–22 September 2005; pp. 299–306.

80. Szklarczyk, D.; Morris, J.H.; Cook, H.; Kuhn, M.; Wyder, S.; Simonovic, M.; Santos, A.; Doncheva, N.T.; Roth, A.; Bork, P.; et al. The STRING database in 2017: Quality-Controlled protein–protein association networks, made broadly accessible. *Nucleic Acids Res.* **2017**, *45*, D362–D368. [CrossRef] [PubMed]

81. Shannon, P.; Markiel, A.; Ozier, O.; Baliga, N.S.; Wang, J.T.; Ramage, D.; Amin, N.; Schwikowski, B.; Ideker, T. Cytoscape: A software Environment for integrated models of biomolecular interaction networks. *Genome Res.* **2003**, *13*, 2498–2504. [CrossRef]

82. Ritz, A.; Poirel, C.L.; Tegge, A.N.; Sharp, N.; Simmons, K.; Powell, A.; Kale, S.D.; Murali, T. Pathways on demand: Automated reconstruction of human signaling networks. *NPJ Syst. Biol. Appl.* **2016**, *2*, 16002. [CrossRef]

83. Rodríguez, Y.; Alejo, C.; Alejo, I.; Viguria, A. ANIMO, framework to simplify the real-time distributed communication. In *Management of Cyber Physical Objects in the Future Internet of Things*; Guerrieri, A., Loscri, V., Rovella, A., Fortino, G., Eds.; Springer: Berlin, Germany, 2016; pp. 77–92.

84. Kaushik, A.C. Logisim Operon Circuits. *IJSER* **2013**, *4*, 5.

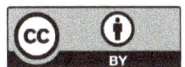

MDPI

St. Alban-Anlage 66

4052 Basel

Switzerland

Tel. +41 61 683 77 34

Fax +41 61 302 89 18

www.mdpi.com

Marine Drugs Editorial Office

E-mail: marinedrugs@mdpi.com

www.mdpi.com/journal/marinedrugs